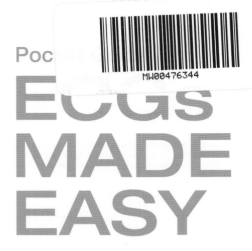

Pocket Guide

ECGs
MADE
EASY

Barbara Aehlert, MSEd, BSPA, RN

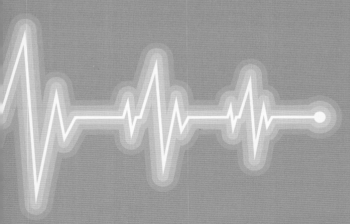

ELSEVIER

Sixth Edition

ELSEVIER

3251 Riverport Lane
St. Louis, Missouri 63043

POCKET GUIDE FOR ECGs MADE EASY,
SIXTH EDITION   ISBN: 978-0-323-40129-6

Notices

Knowledge and best practice in this field are constantly changing. As new research and experience broaden our understanding, changes in research methods, professional practices, or medical treatment may become necessary.

Practitioners and researchers must always rely on their own experience and knowledge in evaluating and using any information, methods, compounds, or experiments described herein. In using such information or methods they should be mindful of their own safety and the safety of others, including parties for whom they have a professional responsibility.

With respect to any drug or pharmaceutical products identified, readers are advised to check the most current information provided (i) on procedures featured or (ii) by the manufacturer of each product to be administered, to verify the recommended dose or formula, the method and duration of administration, and contraindications. It is the responsibility of practitioners, relying on their own experience and knowledge of their patients, to make diagnoses, to determine dosages and the best treatment for each individual patient, and to take all appropriate safety precautions.

To the fullest extent of the law, neither the Publisher nor the authors, contributors, or editors, assume any liability for any injury and/or damage to persons or property as a matter of products liability, negligence or otherwise, or from any use or operation of any methods, products, instructions, or ideas contained in the material herein.

Senior Content Strategist: Sandy Clark
Content Development Manager: Lisa Newton
Senior Content Development Specialist: Laura Selkirk/Melissa Kinsey
Publishing Services Manager: Deepthi Unni
Project Manager: Janish Ashwin Paul
Design Direction: Brian Salisbury

Printed in China

Last digit is the print number: 9 8 7 6 5 4 3

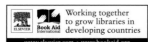

Working together
to grow libraries in
developing countries

www.elsevier.com • www.bookaid.org

Preface

This pocket guide is a handy, easy-to-use manual for interpretation of basic dysrhythmias. It's intended to accompany the sixth edition of the *ECGs Made Easy* textbook. In this reference, we've included a brief description of most of the rhythms discussed in the textbook. Each description is presented with a summary of rhythm characteristics and a sample rhythm strip.

All rhythm strips were recorded in lead II unless otherwise noted. Signs and symptoms associated with each rhythm, as well as treatment options, are outlined in the *ECGs Made Easy* textbook. We've made every attempt to provide information consistent with the current literature, including the latest resuscitation guidelines.

I hope you find this pocket guide helpful, and I wish you success in your studies and work.

Best regards,
Barbara Aehlert

Acknowledgments

I would like to thank the manuscript reviewers for *ECGs Made Easy,* sixth edition. Their comments and suggestions helped in rewriting, reorganizing, and clarifying this content.

I would also like to thank the following healthcare professionals, who provided many of the rhythm strips used in this book: Andrew Baird, CEP; James Bratcher; Joanna Burgan, CEP; Holly Button, CEP; Gretchen Chalmers, CEP; Thomas Cole, CEP; Brent Haines, CEP; Paul Honeywell, CEP; Timothy Klatt, RN; Bill Loughran, RN; Andrea Lowrey, RN; Joe Martinez, CEP; Stephanos Orphanidis, CEP; Jason Payne, CEP; Steve Ruehs, CEP; Patty Seneski, RN; David Stockton, CEP; Jason Stodghill, CEP; Dionne Socie, CEP; Kristina Tellez, CEP; and Fran Wojculewicz, RN.

Barbara Aehlert, MSEd, BSPA, RN, has been a registered nurse for more than 40 years, with clinical experience in medical/surgical nursing, critical care nursing, prehospital education, and nursing education. Barbara is an active CPR and ACLS instructor with a special interest in teaching basic dysrhythmia recognition and ACLS to nurses and paramedics.

Contents

Anatomy and Physiology

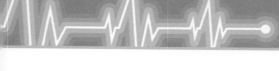

LOCATION AND SURFACES OF THE HEART

The heart is a hollow muscular organ that lies in the space between the lungs (ie, the mediastinum) in the middle of the chest. It sits behind the sternum and just above the diaphragm (Fig. 1.1). About two-thirds of the heart lies to the left of the midline of the sternum. The remaining third lies to the right of the sternum.

The base, or posterior surface of the heart, is formed by the left atrium, a small portion of the right atrium, and proximal portions of the superior and inferior venae cavae and the pulmonary veins. The front (anterior) surface of the heart lies behind the sternum and costal

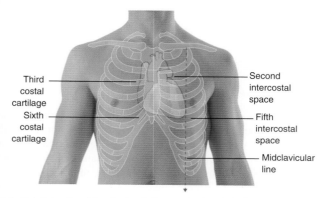

Third costal cartilage

Sixth costal cartilage

Second intercostal space

Fifth intercostal space

Midclavicular line

Fig. 1.1 Anterior view of the chest wall of a man showing skeletal structures and the surface projection of the heart. (From Drake R, Vogl AW, Mitchell AWM: *Gray's anatomy for students,* ed 3, New York, 2015, Churchill Livingstone.)

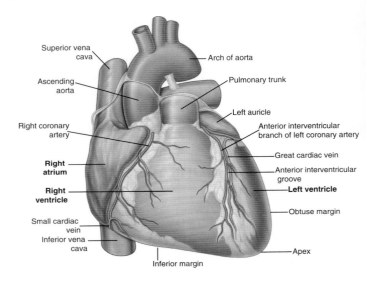

Fig. 1.2 The anterior surface of the heart. (From Drake R, Vogl AW, Mitchell AWM: *Gray's anatomy for students,* ed 3, New York, 2015, Churchill Livingstone.)

cartilages. It is formed by portions of the right atrium and the left and right ventricles (Fig. 1.2). The heart's apex, or lower portion, is formed by the tip of the left ventricle. The apex lies just above the diaphragm at about the level of the fifth intercostal space in the midclavicular line.

STRUCTURE OF THE HEART

Layers of the Heart Wall

The walls of the heart are made up of three tissue layers: the endocardium, myocardium, and epicardium. The heart's innermost layer, the *endocardium*, is made up of a thin, smooth layer of epithelium and connective tissue, and lines the heart's inner chambers, valves, chordae tendineae (tendinous cords), and papillary muscles. The endocardium is continuous with the innermost layer of the arteries, veins, and capillaries of the body, thereby creating a continuous, closed circulatory system. The *myocardium* (middle layer) is a thick, muscular layer that consists of cardiac muscle fibers (cells) responsible for the

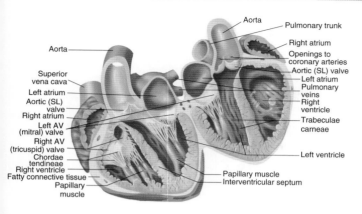

Fig. 1.3 Interior of the heart. This illustration shows the heart as it would appear if it were cut along a frontal plane and opened like a book. The front portion of the heart lies to the reader's right; the back portion of the heart lies to the reader's left. The four chambers of the heart—two atria and two ventricles—are easily seen. *AV*, atrioventricular; *SL*, semilunar. (From Patton KT, Thibodeau GA: *Anatomy & physiology,* ed 9, St. Louis, 2016, Mosby.)

pumping action of the heart. The heart's outermost layer is called the *epicardium*. The epicardium contains blood capillaries, lymph capillaries, nerve fibers, and fat. The main coronary arteries lie on the epicardial surface of the heart.

Heart Chambers

The heart has four chambers (Fig. 1.3). The two upper chambers are the right and left atria. The purpose of the atria is to receive blood. The right atrium receives blood low in oxygen from the superior vena cava (which carries blood from the head and upper extremities), the inferior vena cava (which carries blood from the lower body), and the coronary sinus (which is the largest vein that drains the heart). The left atrium receives freshly oxygenated blood from the lungs via the right and left pulmonary veins.

The heart's two lower chambers are the right and left ventricles. Their purpose is to pump blood. The right ventricle pumps blood to the lungs. The left ventricle pumps blood out to the body.

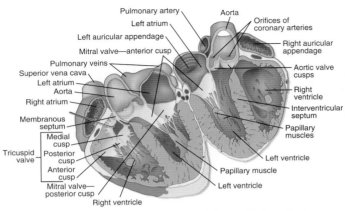

Fig. 1.4 Drawing of a heart split perpendicular to the interventricular septum to illustrate the anatomic relationships of the leaflets of the atrioventricular and aortic valves. (Koeppen BM, Stanton BA: *Berne & Levy physiology*, ed 6, St. Louis, 2010, Mosby.)

Heart Valves

There are four one-way valves in the heart: two sets of atrioventricular (AV) valves and two sets of semilunar (SL) valves (Fig. 1.4). The valves open and close in a specific sequence and assist in producing the pressure gradient needed between the chambers to ensure a smooth flow of blood through the heart and prevent the backflow of blood.

AV valves separate the atria from the ventricles. The tricuspid valve is the AV valve that lies between the right atrium and right ventricle. It consists of three separate cusps or flaps. It is larger in diameter and thinner than the mitral valve. The mitral (or bicuspid) valve has only two cusps. It lies between the left atrium and left ventricle.

The pulmonic and aortic valves are SL valves. The SL valves prevent backflow of blood from the aorta and pulmonary arteries into the ventricles. The SL valves have three cusps shaped like half-moons. The openings of the SL valves are smaller than the openings of the AV valves, and the flaps of the SL valves are smaller and thicker than the AV valves.

Heart sounds occur because of vibrations in the tissues of the heart caused by the closing of the heart's valves. Vibrations are created as blood flow is suddenly increased or slowed with the contraction and relaxation of the heart chambers and with the opening and closing of the valves. The first heart sound ("lubb") occurs during ventricular contraction when the tricuspid and mitral (AV) valves close. The second heart sound ("dupp") occurs during ventricular relaxation when the pulmonic and aortic (SL) valves close.

THE HEART'S BLOOD SUPPLY

The coronary circulation consists of coronary arteries and veins. The main coronary arteries lie on the outer (epicardial) surface of the heart. The three major coronary arteries include the left anterior descending (LAD) artery, circumflex (Cx) artery, and the right coronary artery (RCA) (Fig. 1.5; Table 1.1). A person is said to have coronary artery disease (CAD) if there is more than 50% diameter narrowing (ie, stenosis) in one or more of these vessels.

The coronary (cardiac) veins travel alongside the arteries. The coronary sinus is the largest vein that drains the heart. It lies in the groove separating the atria from the ventricles. Blood that has passed through the myocardial capillaries is drained by the branches of the cardiac veins that join the coronary sinus.

Acute Coronary Syndromes

The term *acute coronary syndrome* (ACS) refers to a set of distinct conditions caused by a similar sequence of pathologic events involving an abrupt reduction in coronary artery blood flow. This sequence of events produces conditions ranging from myocardial ischemia or injury to death (ie, necrosis) of the heart muscle. The usual cause of an ACS is the rupture of an atherosclerotic plaque. *Arteriosclerosis* is a chronic disease of the arterial system characterized by abnormal thickening and hardening of the vessel walls. *Atherosclerosis* is a form of arteriosclerosis in which the thickening and hardening of the vessel walls are caused by a buildup of fat-like deposits (eg, plaque) in the inner lining of large- and middle-sized muscular arteries. As the fatty deposits build up, the opening of the artery slowly narrows, and blood flow to the muscle decreases (Fig. 1.6). The complete blockage of a coronary artery may cause a heart attack or *myocardial infarction* (MI).

Angina pectoris is chest discomfort or other related symptoms that occur suddenly when the increased oxygen demand of the heart temporarily exceeds its blood supply. Angina is not a disease. Rather, it is a symptom of myocardial ischemia. Angina most often occurs in patients with CAD involving at least one coronary artery. However, it can be present in patients with normal coronary arteries. Angina also occurs in people with uncontrolled high blood pressure or valvular heart disease.

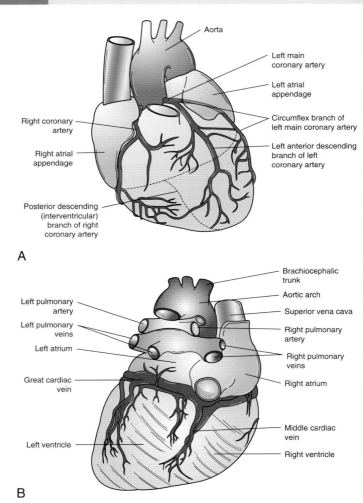

A

B

Fig. 1.5 Coronary arteries supplying the heart. The right coronary artery supplies the right atrium, ventricle, and posterior aspect of the left ventricle in most individuals. The left coronary artery divides into the left anterior descending and circumflex arteries, which perfuse the left ventricle. A, Anterior view. B, Posterior view. (From Copstead-Kirkhorn L, Banasik JL: *Pathophysiology,* ed 5, Philadelphia, 2013, Elsevier.)

TABLE 1.1	Coronary Arteries	
Coronary Artery	**Portion of Myocardium Supplied**	**Portion of Conduction System Supplied**
Right	<ul><li>Right atrium</li><li>Right ventricle</li><li>Inferior surface of left ventricle (about 85%)*</li><li>Posterior surface of left ventricle (85%)*</li></ul>	<ul><li>Sinoatrial (SA) node (in about 60%)*</li><li>Atrioventricular (AV) bundle (85% to 90%)*</li></ul>
Left anterior descending	<ul><li>Anterior surface of left ventricle</li><li>Part of lateral surface of left ventricle</li><li>Anterior two thirds of interventricular septum</li></ul>	<ul><li>Most of right bundle branch</li><li>Part of left bundle branch</li></ul>
Circumflex	<ul><li>Left atrium</li><li>Part of lateral surface of left ventricle</li><li>Inferior surface of left ventricle (about 15%)*</li><li>Posterior surface of left ventricle (15%)*</li></ul>	<ul><li>SA node (about 40%)*</li><li>AV bundle (10% to 15%)*</li></ul>

*Of population.

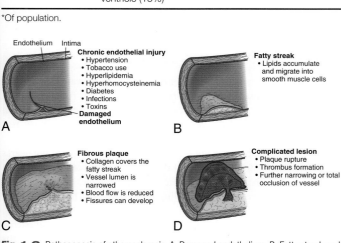

Fig. 1.6 Pathogenesis of atherosclerosis. A, Damaged endothelium. B, Fatty streak and lipid core formation. C, Fibrous plaque. Raised plaques are visible: some are yellow, others are white. D, Complicated lesion: thrombus is red, collagen is blue. Plaque is complicated by red thrombus deposition. (From Lewis, S, Dirksen S, Heitkemper M, Bucher L: *Medical-surgical nursing: Assessment and management of clinical problems,* ed 9, St. Louis, 2014, Mosby.)

Chest discomfort associated with myocardial ischemia usually begins in the central or left chest then radiates to the arm (especially the little finger [ulnar] side of the left arm), the wrist, the jaw, the epigastrium, the left shoulder, or between the shoulder blades.

Ischemia can occur because of increased myocardial oxygen demand (ie, demand ischemia), reduced myocardial oxygen supply (ie, supply ischemia), or both. If the cause of the ischemia is not reversed and blood flow restored to the affected area of the heart muscle, ischemia may lead to cellular injury and, ultimately, infarction. Ischemia can quickly resolve by reducing the heart's oxygen demand, by resting or slowing the heart rate with medications such as beta-blockers, or by increasing blood flow by dilating the coronary arteries with drugs such as nitroglycerin.

Injured myocardial cells are still alive but will die (ie, *infarct*) if the ischemia is not quickly corrected. An MI occurs when blood flow to the heart muscle stops or is suddenly decreased long enough to cause cell death. If the blocked coronary vessel can be quickly opened to restore blood flow and oxygen to the injured area, no tissue death occurs. Methods to restore blood flow may include giving clot-busting drugs (ie, fibrinolytics), performing coronary angioplasty, or performing a coronary artery bypass graft, among others.

THE HEART'S NERVE SUPPLY

Both divisions of the autonomic nervous system innervate fibers to the heart. The sympathetic division prepares the body to function under stress (ie, the "fight-or-flight" response). The parasympathetic division conserves and restores body resources (ie, the "feed-and-breed" or "rest and digest" response).

Sympathetic (accelerator) nerves innervate specific areas of the heart's electrical system, atrial muscle, and the ventricular myocardium. When sympathetic nerves are stimulated, the neurotransmitters norepinephrine and epinephrine are released resulting in an increased heart rate, force of contraction, conduction velocity, blood pressure, and cardiac output.

Parasympathetic (inhibitory) nerve fibers innervate the sinoatrial (SA) node, atrial muscle, and the AV bundle of the heart by the vagus nerves. Acetylcholine is a chemical messenger (neurotransmitter) released when parasympathetic nerves are stimulated. Parasympathetic stimulation slows the rate of discharge of the SA node, slows conduction through the AV node, decreases the strength of atrial contraction, and can cause a small decrease in the force of ventricular contraction.

THE HEART AS A PUMP

The right and left sides of the heart are separated by an internal wall of connective tissue called a *septum*. The *interatrial septum* separates the right and left atria. The *interventricular septum* separates the right and left ventricles. The septa separate the heart into two functional pumps. The right atrium and right ventricle make up one pump. The left atrium and left ventricle make up the other (Fig. 1.7).

The right side of the heart is a low-pressure system whose job is to pump unoxygenated blood from the body to and through the lungs to the left side of the heart. This is called the *pulmonary circulation*. The job of the left side of the heart is to receive oxygenated blood from the lungs and pump it out to the rest of the body. This is called the *systemic circulation*. Blood is carried from the heart to the organs of the body through arteries, arterioles, and capillaries. Blood is returned to the right side of the heart through venules and veins.

Cardiac Cycle

The cardiac cycle refers to a repetitive pumping process that includes all of the events associated with blood flow through the heart. The cycle has

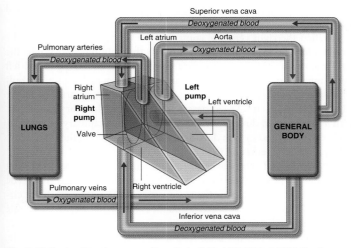

Fig. 1.7 The heart has two pumps. (From Drake R, Vogl AW, Mitchell AWM: *Gray's anatomy for students,* ed 3, New York, 2015, Churchill Livingstone.)

two phases for each heart chamber: systole and diastole. Systole is the period during which the chamber contracts and blood is ejected. *Systole* includes contraction of both atrial and ventricular muscle. *Diastole* is the period of relaxation during which the chambers are allowed to fill. The myocardium receives its fresh supply of oxygenated blood from the coronary arteries during ventricular diastole.

During the cardiac cycle, the pressure within each chamber of the heart rises in systole and falls in diastole. The heart's valves ensure that blood flows in the proper direction. Blood flows from one heart chamber to another from higher to lower pressure. These pressure relationships depend on the careful timing of contractions. The heart's conduction system provides the necessary timing of events between atrial and ventricular systole.

Blood from the tissues of the head, neck, and upper extremities is emptied into the superior vena cava. Blood from the lower body is returned to the inferior vena cava. During atrial diastole, blood from the superior and inferior vena cavae and the coronary sinus enters the right atrium (Fig. 1.8). The right atrium fills and distends. This pushes the tricuspid valve open and the right ventricle fills.

The left atrium receives oxygenated blood from the four pulmonary veins (two from the right lung and two from the left lung). The flaps of the mitral valve open as the left atrium fills. This allows blood to flow into the left ventricle. As the ventricles contract, blood is propelled through the systemic and pulmonary circulation and toward the atria.

When the right ventricle contracts, the tricuspid valve closes. The right ventricle expels the blood through the pulmonic valve into the pulmonary trunk. The pulmonary trunk divides into a right and left pulmonary artery, each of which carries blood to one lung (ie, the pulmonary circuit). Blood flows through the pulmonary arteries to the lungs. Blood low in oxygen passes through the pulmonary capillaries. There it comes in direct contact with the alveolar-capillary membrane, where oxygen and carbon dioxide are exchanged. Blood then flows into the pulmonary veins and then to the left atrium.

When the left ventricle contracts, the mitral valve closes to prevent backflow of blood. Blood leaves the left ventricle through the aortic valve to the aorta, which is the main vessel of the systemic arterial circulation. Blood is distributed throughout the body (ie, the systemic circuit) through the aorta and its branches. Blood continues to move in one direction because pressure pushes it from the high-pressure (ie, arterial) side, and valves in the veins prevent backflow on the lower pressure (ie, venous) side as blood returns to the heart.

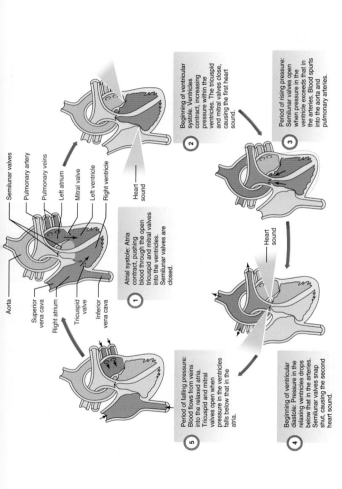

Fig. 1.8 Blood flow through the heart during the cardiac cycle. (From Solomon E: *Introduction to human anatomy and physiology*, ed 4, St. Louis, 2016, Saunders.)

Box 1.1	Signs and Symptoms of Decreased Cardiac Output

- Acute changes in blood pressure
- Acute changes in mental status
- Cold, clammy skin
- Color changes in the skin and mucous membranes
- Crackles (rales)
- Dyspnea
- Dysrhythmias
- Fatigue
- Orthopnea
- Restlessness

Blood Pressure

The mechanical activity of the heart is reflected by the pulse and blood pressure. *Blood pressure* is the force exerted by the circulating blood volume on the walls of the arteries. The volume of blood in the arteries is directly related to arterial blood pressure. Blood pressure is equal to cardiac output × peripheral resistance. *Peripheral resistance* is the resistance to the flow of blood determined by blood vessel diameter and the tone of the vascular musculature. Blood pressure is affected by conditions or medications that alter peripheral resistance or cardiac output.

Cardiac output is the amount of blood pumped into the aorta each minute by the heart. It is defined as the *stroke volume*, which is the amount of blood ejected from a ventricle with each heartbeat, multiplied by the heart rate. In a healthy average adult, the cardiac output at rest is about 5 L/min. The percentage of blood pumped out of a ventricle with each contraction is called the *ejection fraction*. Ejection fraction is used as a measure of ventricular function. A normal ejection fraction is between 50% and 65%. Signs and symptoms of decreased cardiac output appear in Box 1.1.

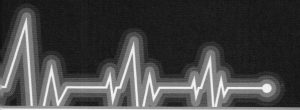

Basic Electrophysiology

2

CARDIAC CELLS

Types of Cardiac Cells

In general, cardiac cells have either a mechanical (ie, contractile) or an electrical (ie, pacemaker) function. *Myocardial cells* contain contractile filaments. When these cells are electrically stimulated, these filaments slide together and cause the myocardial cell to contract. These myocardial cells form the thin muscular layer of the atrial walls and the thicker muscular layer of the ventricular walls (ie, the myocardium). These cells do not normally generate electrical impulses, and they rely on pacemaker cells for this function.

Pacemaker cells are specialized cells of the electrical conduction system. Pacemaker cells are also known as *conducting cells* or *automatic cells*. They are able to form electrical impulses spontaneously and can alter the speed of electrical conduction.

Properties of Cardiac Cells

The ability of cardiac pacemaker cells to create an electrical impulse without stimulation from another source is called *automaticity*. *Excitability* (ie, irritability) is the ability of cardiac muscle cells to respond to an external stimulus, such as that from a chemical, mechanical, or electrical source. *Conductivity* is the ability of a cardiac cell to receive an electrical impulse and conduct it to an adjoining cardiac cell. All cardiac cells possess this characteristic. *Contractility* (ie, inotropy) is the ability of myocardial cells to shorten, thereby causing cardiac muscle contraction in response to an electrical stimulus. The heart normally contracts in response to an impulse that begins in the sinoatrial (SA) node.

CARDIAC ACTION POTENTIAL

Human body fluids contain *electrolytes*, which are elements or compounds that break into charged particles (*ions*) when melted or dissolved in water or another solvent. Differences in the composition of ions between the intracellular and extracellular fluid compartments are important for normal body function, including the activity of the heart.

Electrolytes are quickly moved from one side of the cell membrane to the other by means of pumps. These pumps require energy in the form of adenosine triphosphate (ATP) when movement occurs against a concentration gradient. The energy expended by the cells to move electrolytes across the cell membrane creates a flow of current. This flow of current is expressed in volts. Voltage appears on an electrocardiogram (ECG) as spikes or waveforms.

The *action potential* of a cardiac cell reflects the rapid sequence of voltage changes across the cell membrane during the electrical cardiac cycle. The configuration of the action potential varies depending on the location, size, and function of the cardiac cell.

There are two main types of action potentials in the heart (Fig. 2.1). The first type, the fast response action potential, occurs in

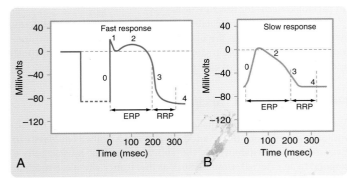

Fig. 2.1 Action potentials of fast-response (A) and slow-response (B) cardiac fibers. The phases of the action potentials are labeled. The effective refractory period (ERP) and the relative refractory period (RRP) are labeled. Note that when compared to fast-response fibers, the resting potential of slow fibers is less negative, the upstroke (phase 0) of the action potential is less steep, the amplitude of the action potential is smaller, phase 1 is absent, and the RRP extends well into phase 4 after the fibers have fully repolarized. (From Koeppen BM, Stanton BA: *Berne & Levy physiology,* ed 6, St. Louis, 2010, Mosby.)

normal atrial and ventricular myocardial cells and in the Purkinje fibers, which are specialized conducting fibers in both ventricles that conduct electrical impulses through the heart. The second type of cardiac action potential, the slow response action potential, occurs in the heart's normal pacemaker (ie, the SA node) and in the atrioventricular (AV) node, which is the specialized conducting tissue that carries an electrical impulse from the atria to the ventricles.

REFRACTORY PERIODS

Refractoriness is a term used to describe the period of recovery that cells need after being discharged before they are able to respond to a stimulus. During the *absolute refractory period* (ARP), the cell will not respond to further stimulation within itself (Fig. 2.2). This means that the myocardial working cells cannot contract and the cells of the electrical conduction system cannot conduct an electrical impulse, no matter how strong the internal electrical stimulus.

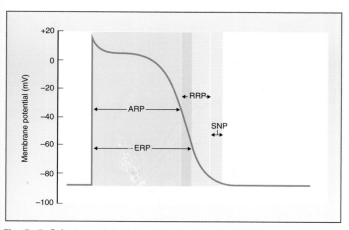

Fig. 2.2 Refractory periods of the ventricular action potential. Refractory periods of the ventricular action potential. The effective refractory period (ERP) includes the absolute refractory period (ARP) and the first half of the relative refractory period (RRP). The RRP begins when the absolute refractory period ends and includes the last portion of the ERP. The supernormal period (SNP) begins when the RRP ends. (From Costanzo LS: *Physiology,* ed 5, Philadelphia, 2014, Saunders.)

The *relative refractory period* (RRP) begins at the end of the ARP and ends when the cell membrane is almost fully repolarized. During the RRP, some cardiac cells have repolarized to their threshold potential and thus can be stimulated to respond (ie, depolarize) to a stronger-than-normal stimulus. The *effective refractory period* includes the ARP and the first half of the RRP.

A *supernormal* period follows the RRP. A weaker-than-normal stimulus can cause cardiac cells to depolarize during this period. Because the cell is more excitable than normal, dysrhythmias can develop during this period.

CONDUCTION SYSTEM

Fig. 2.3 shows the heart's conduction system. A summary of the conduction system is shown in Table 2.1.

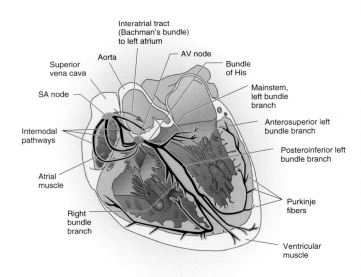

Fig. 2.3 Conduction pathways through the heart. (From Boron WF: *Medical physiology,* ed 2 [updated edition], Philadelphia, 2011, Saunders.)

TABLE **2.1**	Cardiac Conduction System		
Structure	**Location**	**Function**	**Intrinsic Pacemaker (beats/min)**
Sinoatrial (SA) node	Right atrial wall just inferior to opening of superior vena cava	Primary pacemaker; initiates impulse that is normally conducted throughout the left and right atria	60 to 100
Atrioventricular (AV) node	Floor of the right atrium immediately behind the tricuspid valve and near the opening of the coronary sinus	Receives impulse from SA node and delays relay of the impulse to the bundle of His, allowing time for the atria to empty their contents into the ventricles before the onset of ventricular contraction	
Bundle of His (AV bundle)	Superior portion of interventricular septum	Receives impulse from AV node and relays it to right and left bundle branches	40 to 60
Right and left bundle branches	Interventricular septum	Receives impulse from bundle of His and relays it to Purkinje fibers	
Purkinje fibers	Ventricular myocardium	Receives impulse from bundle branches and relays it to ventricular myocardium	20 to 40

CAUSES OF DYSRHYTHMIAS

Dysrhythmias result from disorders of impulse formation, disorders of impulse conduction, or both.

Disorders of Impulse Formation

Abnormal Automaticity

Abnormal automaticity is a condition in which one of the following occurs: (1) Cardiac cells not normally associated with a pacemaker function begin to depolarize spontaneously *or* (2) a pacemaker site other than the SA node increases its firing rate beyond that which is considered normal.

Triggered Activity

Triggered activity results from abnormal electrical impulses that sometimes occur during repolarization, when cells are normally quiet. These abnormal electrical impulses are called *afterdepolarizations*. Triggered activity requires a stimulus to begin depolarization. It occurs when pacemaker cells from a site other than the SA node and myocardial working cells depolarize more than once after being stimulated by a single impulse.

Disorders of Impulse Conduction

Conduction Blocks

Blocks of impulse conduction may be partial or complete. A partial conduction block may be slowed or intermittent. In slowed conduction, all impulses are conducted, but it takes longer than normal to do so. When an intermittent block occurs, some (but not all) impulses are conducted. When a complete block exists, no impulses are conducted through the affected area. Examples of rhythms associated with disturbances in conduction include AV blocks.

Reentry

An impulse normally spreads through the heart only once after it is initiated by pacemaker cells. *Reentry* is the spread of an impulse through tissue already stimulated by that same impulse. Reentry requires the following three conditions: (1) An area of unidirectional conduction block, (2) an area of delayed conduction, and (3) an area of unexcitable tissue. When reentry occurs, an electrical impulse is delayed, blocked, or both in one or more areas of the conduction system while the impulse is conducted normally through the rest of the conduction system. This results in the delayed electrical impulse entering cardiac cells that have just been depolarized by the normally conducted impulse.

THE ELECTROCARDIOGRAM

An ECG machine functions as a voltmeter, detecting and recording the changes in voltage (ie, action potentials) generated by depolarization and repolarization of the heart's cells. The voltage changes are displayed as specific waveforms and complexes (Fig. 2.4).

ECG monitoring may be used for the following purposes:
- To monitor a patient's heart rate
- To evaluate the effects of disease or injury on heart function
- To evaluate pacemaker function

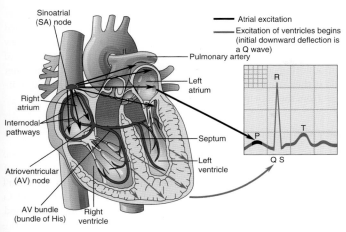

Fig. 2.4 Schematic drawing of the conducting system of the heart. An impulse normally is generated in the sinoatrial node and travels through the atria to the atrioventricular (AV) node, down the bundle of His and Purkinje fibers, and to the ventricular myocardium. Recording of the depolarizing and repolarizing currents in the heart with electrodes on the surface of the body produces characteristic waveforms. (From Copstead-Kirkhorn LE, Banasik JL: *Pathophysiology,* ed 5, St. Louis, 2013, Saunders.)

- To evaluate the response to medications (eg, antiarrhythmics)
- To obtain a baseline recording before, during, and after a medical procedure
- To evaluate for signs of myocardial ischemia, injury, and infarction
  The ECG *can* provide information about the following:
- The orientation of the heart in the chest
- Conduction disturbances
- Electrical effects of medications and electrolytes
- The mass of cardiac muscle
- The presence of ischemic damage
  The ECG does *not* provide information about the mechanical (contractile) condition of the myocardium. To evaluate the effectiveness of the heart's mechanical activity, the patient's pulse and blood pressure are assessed.

Electrodes

An *electrode* is an adhesive pad containing a conductive substance. When the electrode is applied to a patient's skin, the conductive medium at the center of the pad conducts skin surface voltage changes through the attached wires to a cardiac monitor. Electrodes are applied at specific locations on the patient's chest wall and extremities to view the heart's electrical activity from selected angles and planes. One end of a monitoring cable, or *lead wire*, is attached to the electrode. The other end of the cable is attached to an ECG machine. The cable conducts current from the patient to the cardiac monitor.

Leads

A *lead* is a record (ie, tracing) of electrical activity between two electrodes. Each lead records the *average* current flow at a specific time in a portion of the heart. Leads allow viewing the heart's electrical activity in two different planes: frontal (coronal) and horizontal (transverse). A 12-lead ECG provides views of the heart in both the frontal and horizontal planes and views the surfaces of the left ventricle from 12 different angles (Fig. 2.5).

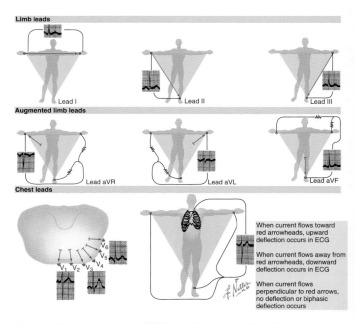

Fig. 2.5 The electrocardiogram (ECG) leads. (From Runge MS: *Netter's cardiology*, ed 2, Philadelphia, 2010, Saunders.)

A summary of the standard limb leads can be found in Table 2.2, a summary of the augmented leads appears in Table 2.3, and a summary of the chest leads appears in Table 2.4.

Right Chest Leads

Other chest leads that are not part of a standard 12-lead ECG may be used to view specific surfaces of the heart. Right chest leads are used to evaluate the right ventricle. The placement of right chest leads is identical to the placement of the standard chest leads except that it is done on the right side of the chest (Fig. 2.6). If time does not permit obtaining all of the right chest leads, the lead of choice is V_4R.

Posterior Chest Leads

On a standard 12-lead ECG, no leads look directly at the posterior surface of the heart. Additional chest leads may be used for this purpose. These leads are placed further left and toward the back. All of the leads are placed on the same horizontal line as V_4 through V_6. Lead V_7 is placed at the posterior axillary line. Lead V_8 is placed at the angle of the scapula (ie, the posterior scapular line) and lead V_9 is placed over the left border of spine (Fig. 2.7).

Ambulatory Cardiac Monitoring

External ambulatory cardiac monitoring, also known as *ambulatory electrocardiographic (AECG) monitoring,* is a noninvasive diagnostic

TABLE 2.2	Standard Limb Leads		
Lead	Positive Electrode	Negative Electrode	Heart Surface Viewed
I	Left arm	Right arm	Lateral
II	Left leg	Right arm	Inferior
III	Left leg	Left arm	Inferior

TABLE 2.3	Augmented Leads	
Lead	Positive Electrode	Heart Surface Viewed
aVR	Right arm	None
aVL	Left arm	Lateral
aVF	Left leg	Inferior

TABLE **2.4**	Chest Leads	
Lead	Positive Electrode Position	Heart Surface Viewed
V_1	Right side of sternum, fourth intercostal space	Interventricular septum
V_2	Left side of sternum, fourth intercostal space	Interventricular septum
V_3	Midway between V_2 and V_4	Anterior surface
V_4	Left midclavicular line, fifth intercostal space	Anterior surface
V_5	Left anterior axillary line; same level as V_4	Lateral surface
V_6	Left midaxillary line; fifth intercostal space	Lateral surface

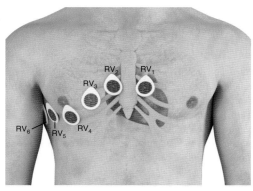

Fig. 2.6 Electrode locations for recording a right chest electrocardiogram (ECG). (From Roberts JR [Ed.]: *Roberts and Hedges' clinical procedures in emergency medicine*, ed 6, Philadelphia, 2014, Saunders.)

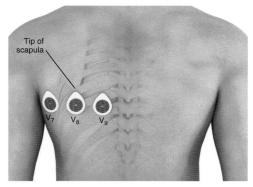

Fig. 2.7 Electrode locations for left posterior chest lead placement. (From Roberts JR [Ed.]: *Roberts and Hedges' clinical procedures in emergency medicine*, ed 6, Philadelphia, 2014, Saunders.)

tool used to monitor the patient's cardiac rhythm while performing his or her daily activities. Examples of indications for AECG monitoring include the following:

- To determine the association between a patient's symptoms (eg, dizziness, palpitations, near syncope, shortness of breath, chest pain, fatigue) and cardiac rhythm disturbances
- To detect myocardial ischemia and to evaluate the efficacy of anti-ischemic medications in patients with coronary artery disease
- To assess the patient's risk of dysrhythmias after a myocardial infarction; for patients with heart failure, hypertrophic cardiomyopathy, diabetic neuropathy, systemic hypertension, or valvular heart disease; for patients receiving hemodialysis; and for the preoperative evaluation of patients and after cardiac operations
- To assess the efficacy of medications on the cardiac conduction system, the patient's cardiac rhythm, or both
- To aid in correlating patient symptoms with dysrhythmias and evaluating symptomatic patients for pacemaker implantation
- To assess the function of implanted devices, such as a pacemaker or an implantable cardioverter-defibrillator
- To assess the efficacy of ablation procedures

A conventional Holter monitor is a battery-powered continuous AECG recorder used for 24 hours up to a maximum of 72 hours to document ECG events likely to occur within this period. Electrodes and lead wires are connected to a portable, lightweight recorder that is attached to the patient and carried with a belt or shoulder strap. Patients are asked to keep a log or diary while the device is in use. Newer Holter monitors permit extended ECG monitoring, typically for 7 to 14 days, using a patch-based system (Fig. 2.8). During extended Holter monitoring, data is recorded continuously and transmitted to a central monitoring station.

Event recorders, also called *intermittent recorders*, may be used for longer periods (generally up to 30 days) to document events that are brief, infrequent, or unlikely to be captured during a 24- to 72-hour period.

Electrocardiography Paper

When you place electrodes on the patient's body and connect them to an ECG, the machine records the voltage (ie, the potential difference)

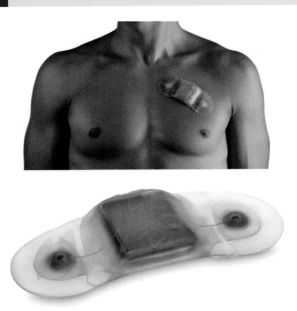

Fig. 2.8 Sample patch-based recording system that allows both acquisition and storage of a single-lead electrocardiogram for 7 to 14 days. (From Krahn AD, Yee R, Skanes AC, Klein GJ: Cardiac monitoring: Short and long term recording. In DP Zipes, & J Jalife [Eds.]: *Cardiac electrophysiology: From cell to bedside,* ed 6, Philadelphia, 2013, Saunders.)

between the electrodes. The needle (or pen) of the ECG moves a specific distance depending on the voltage measured. This recording is made on ECG paper.

ECG paper is graph paper made up of small and large boxes measured in millimeters. The smallest boxes are 1 mm wide and 1 mm high (Fig. 2.9). The horizontal axis of the paper corresponds to time. Time is used to measure the interval between or duration of specific cardiac events, which is stated in seconds.

ECG paper normally records at a constant speed of 25 mm/sec. Thus, each horizontal unit (ie, each 1-mm box) represents 0.04 second (25 mm/sec × 0.04 second = 1 mm). The lines after every five small boxes on the paper are heavier. The heavier lines indicate one large box. Because each large box is the width of five small boxes, a large box represents 0.20 second. Five large boxes, each consisting of five small boxes,

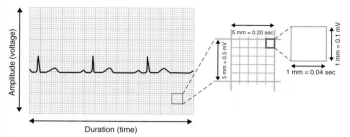

Fig. 2.9 Electrocardiographic strip showing the markings for measuring amplitude and duration of waveforms, using a standard recording speed of 25 mm/sec. (From Copstead-Kirkhorn LE, Banasik JL: *Pathophysiology,* ed 4, Philadelphia, 2009, Saunders.)

represent 1 second; 15 large boxes equal an interval of 3 seconds; and 30 large boxes represent 6 seconds.

The vertical axis of the graph paper represents the voltage or amplitude of the ECG waveforms or deflections. Voltage is measured in millivolts (mV). Voltage may appear as a positive or negative value, because voltage is a force with direction as well as amplitude. Amplitude is measured in millimeters (mm). The default value for ECG machine calibration is 10 mm/mV. This means that when the ECG machine is properly calibrated, a 1-mV electrical signal produces a deflection that measures exactly 10 mm tall (ie, the height of 10 small boxes). Clinically, the height of a waveform is usually stated in mm rather than in mV.

WAVEFORMS

A *waveform* (ie, a deflection) is movement away from the baseline in a positive (ie, upward) or negative (ie, downward) direction. Each waveform that you see on an ECG is related to a specific electrical event in the heart. Waveforms are named alphabetically, beginning with P, QRS, T, and occasionally U. When electrical activity is not detected, a straight line is recorded. This line is called the *baseline* or *isoelectric line*.

P Wave

The first waveform in the cardiac cycle is the P wave (Fig. 2.10). The beginning of the P wave is recognized as the first abrupt or gradual

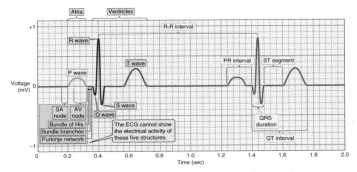

Fig. 2.10 Components of the electrocardiogram (ECG) recording. *AV,* atrioventricular; *SA,* sinoatrial. (From Boron WF, Boulpaep EL: *Medical physiology,* ed 2 updated edition, Philadelphia, 2011, Saunders.)

movement away from the baseline; its end is the point at which the waveform returns to the baseline. The P wave represents the spread of the electrical impulse throughout the right and left atria (ie, atrial depolarization). A P wave normally precedes each QRS complex.

QRS Complex

A *complex* consists of several waveforms. The QRS complex consists of the Q wave, R wave, and S wave and represents the spread of the electrical impulse through the ventricles (ie, ventricular depolarization) and the sum of all ventricular muscle cell depolarizations. Ventricular depolarization normally triggers contraction of ventricular tissue. Thus, shortly after the QRS complex begins, the ventricles contract.

A QRS complex normally follows each P wave. One or even two of the three waveforms that make up the QRS complex may not always be present. When it is present, the Q wave is the first downward deflection following the P wave, and it represents depolarization of the interventricular septum. A Q wave is *always* a negative waveform. The Q wave begins when the ECG leaves the isoelectric line in a downward direction and continues until it returns to the isoelectric line. The R wave is the first positive (ie, upright) waveform following the P wave. The S wave is the negative waveform following the R wave. An R wave is *always* positive and an S wave is *always* negative. The R and S waves represent depolarization of the right and left ventricles.

The QRS duration is a measurement of the time required for ventricular depolarization. The width of a QRS complex is most accurately determined when it is viewed and measured in more than one lead. The measurement should be taken from the QRS complex with the longest duration and clearest onset and end. The beginning of the QRS complex is measured from the point where the first wave of the complex begins to deviate from the baseline. The point at which the last wave of the complex begins to level out or distinctly change direction at, above, or below the baseline marks the end of the QRS complex. In adults, the normal duration of the QRS complex is 0.11 second or less. If an electrical impulse does not follow the normal ventricular conduction pathway, it will take longer to depolarize the myocardium. This delay in conduction through the ventricle produces a wider QRS complex.

T Wave

The T wave represents repolarization of both ventricles. The normal T wave is slightly asymmetric: The peak of the waveform is closer to its end than to the beginning, and the first half has a more gradual slope than the second half. The beginning of the T wave is identified as the point where the slope of the ST segment appears to become abruptly or gradually steeper. The T wave ends when it returns to the baseline. The direction of the T wave is normally the same as the QRS complex that precedes it.

U Wave

A U wave is a small waveform that, when seen, follows the T wave. The U wave is thought to represent late repolarization of the Purkinje fibers. However, some cardiologists believe that U waves represent delayed repolarization in areas of the ventricle that undergo late mechanical relaxation or they are simply two-part T waves resulting from a longer action potential duration in some ventricular myocardial cells. Normal U waves are small, round, and symmetric. U waves are most easily seen when the heart rate is slow and are difficult to identify when the rate exceeds 95 beats/min. U waves usually appear in the same direction as the T waves that precede them.

SEGMENTS

A segment is a line between waveforms. It is named by the waveform that precedes or follows it.

PR Segment

The PR segment is part of the PR interval, specifically, the horizontal line between the end of the P wave and the beginning of the QRS complex. The PR segment is normally isoelectric and represents the spread of the electrical impulse from the AV node, through the AV bundle, the right and left bundle branches, and the Purkinje fibers to activate ventricular muscle.

TP Segment

The TP segment is the portion of the ECG tracing between the end of the T wave and the beginning of the following P wave during which there is no electrical activity (Fig. 2.11). When the heart rate is within normal limits, the TP segment is usually isoelectric and used as the reference point from which to estimate the position of the isoelectric line and determine ST-segment displacement.

ST Segment

The portion of the ECG tracing between the QRS complex and the T wave is the ST segment. The term *ST segment* is used regardless of whether the final wave of the QRS complex is an R or an S wave. The ST segment represents the early part of repolarization of the right and left ventricles. The normal ST segment begins at the isoelectric line, extends from the end of the S wave, and curves gradually upward to the beginning of the T wave.

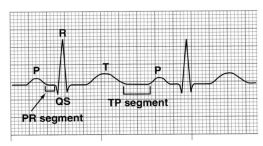

Fig. 2.11 The TP segment is used as the reference point for the isoelectric line if the heart rate is slow enough for the TP segment to be clearly seen.

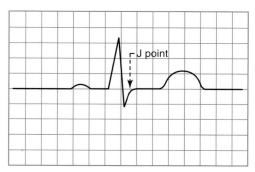

Fig. 2.12 The location of the J point.

The point at which the QRS complex and the ST segment meet is called the *ST junction* or the *J point* (Fig. 2.12). The ST segment is considered elevated if the segment is deviated above the baseline and is considered depressed if the segment deviates below it. When looking for ST-segment elevation or depression, first locate the J point. Next, use the TP segment to estimate the position of the isoelectric line. Then compare the level of the ST segment to the isoelectric line. Deviation is measured as the number of mm of vertical ST segment displacement from the isoelectric line or from the patient's baseline at the J point. Some displacement of the ST segment from the isoelectric line is normal and dependent on age, gender, race, and ECG lead.

INTERVALS

PR Interval

An *interval* is made up of a waveform and a segment. The P wave plus the PR segment equals the PR interval (PRI); thus, the PRI reflects total supraventricular activity.

The PRI is measured from the point where the P wave leaves the baseline to the beginning of the QRS complex. The term *PQ interval* is preferred by some because it is the period actually measured unless a Q wave is absent. The PRI changes with heart rate but normally measures 0.12 to 0.20 second in adults. As the heart rate increases, the duration of the PRI shortens. A PRI is considered *short* if it is less than 0.12 second and *long* if it is more than 0.20 second.

QT Interval

The QT interval is the period from the beginning of the QRS complex to the end of the T wave. It represents total ventricular activity; this is the time from ventricular depolarization (ie, activation) to repolarization (ie, recovery). When measuring the QT interval, first select a lead with the most clearly defined T-wave end. To ensure meaningful comparisons of later tracings, use the same lead for subsequent measurements. In the absence of a Q wave, the QT interval is measured from the beginning of the R wave to the end of the T wave. The term *QT interval* is used regardless of whether the QRS complex begins with a Q wave or an R wave.

The duration of the QT interval varies in accordance with age, gender, and heart rate. As the heart rate increases, the QT interval shortens (i.e., decreases). As the heart rate decreases, the QT interval lengthens (ie, increases). The QT interval is considered short if it is 0.39 second or less and prolonged if it is 0.46 second or longer in women or 0.45 second or longer in men.

R-R and P-P Intervals

The R-R (R wave-to-R wave) and P-P (P wave-to-P wave) intervals are used to determine the rate and rhythmicity (regularity) of a cardiac rhythm. To evaluate the regularity of the ventricular rhythm on a rhythm strip, the interval between two consecutive R waves is measured. The distance between succeeding R-R intervals is measured and compared. If the ventricular rhythm is regular, the R-R intervals will measure the same. To evaluate the rhythmicity of the atrial rhythm, the same procedure is used, but the interval between two consecutive P waves is measured and compared to succeeding P-P intervals.

SYSTEMATIC RHYTHM INTERPRETATION

A systematic approach to rhythm analysis that is consistently applied when analyzing a rhythm strip is essential (Box 2.1). If you do not develop such an approach, you are more likely to miss something important. Begin analyzing the rhythm strip from left to right.

Box **2.1**	Systematic Rhythm Interpretation

1. Assess regularity (atrial and ventricular).
2. Assess rate (atrial and ventricular).
3. Identify and examine waveforms.
4. Assess intervals (eg, PR, QRS, QT) and examine ST segments.
5. Interpret the rhythm and assess its clinical significance.

Assess Regularity

The waveforms on an ECG strip are evaluated for regularity by measuring the distance between the P waves and QRS complexes.

To determine if the ventricular rhythm is regular or irregular, measure the distance between two consecutive R-R intervals. If the ventricular rhythm is regular, the R-R intervals will be equal (measure the same). If the intervals are unequal, the ventricular rhythm is considered irregular. To determine if the atrial rhythm is regular or irregular, follow the same procedure previously described for evaluation of ventricular rhythm but measure the distance between two consecutive P-P intervals (instead of R-R intervals) and compare that distance to the other P-P intervals. The P-P intervals will measure the same if the atrial rhythm is regular. If the intervals are unequal, the atrial rhythm is considered irregular. For accuracy, the R-R or P-P intervals should be evaluated across an entire 6-second rhythm strip.

Assess Rate

Calculation of the heart rate is important because deviations from normal can affect the patient's ability to maintain an adequate blood pressure and cardiac output. Although the atrial rate and ventricular rate are normally the same, the atrial and ventricular rates differ in some dysrhythmias and, therefore, both must be calculated. There are several methods used for calculating heart rate. A discussion of each method follows.

Method 1: 6-Second Method

Most ECG paper is printed with 1-second or 3-second markers on the top or bottom of the paper. On ECG paper, 5 large boxes = 1 second, 15 large boxes = 3 seconds, and 30 large boxes = 6 seconds. To determine the ventricular rate, count the number of complete QRS complexes within a period of 6 seconds and multiply that number by 10 to find the number of complexes in 1 minute (Fig. 2.13). The 6-second method, also called *the rule of 10*, may be used for regular and irregular rhythms. This is the simplest, quickest, and most commonly used method of rate measurement, but it also is the most inaccurate.

Method 2: Large Boxes

The large box method of rate determination is also known as the *rule of 300*. To determine the ventricular rate, count the number of large boxes between an R-R interval and divide into 300 (see Fig. 2.13). To determine the atrial rate, count the number of large boxes between a P-P interval and divide into 300 (Table 2.5). This method is best used if the rhythm is regular; however, it may be used if the rhythm is irregular

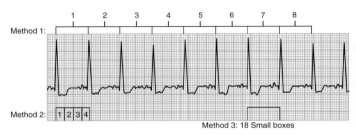

Fig. 2.13 Calculating heart rate. Method 1: Number of R-R intervals in 6 seconds × 10 (eg, 8 × 10 = 80/min). Method 2: Number of large boxes between QRS complexes divided into 300 (eg, 300 divided by 4 = 75/min). Method 3: Number of small boxes between QRS complexes divided into 1,500 (eg, 1,500 divided by 18 = 84/min). (From Clochesy J: *Critical care nursing*, ed 2, Philadelphia, 1996, Saunders.)

TABLE 2.5	Heart Rate Determination Based on the Number of Large Boxes
Number of Large Boxes	**Heart Rate (beats/min)**
1	300
2	150
3	100
4	75
5	60
6	50
7	43
8	38
9	33
10	30

and a rate range (slowest [longest R-R interval] and fastest [shortest R-R interval] rate) is given.

A variation of the large box method is called the *sequence method*. To determine ventricular rate, select an R wave that falls on a dark vertical line. Number the next six consecutive dark vertical lines as follows: 300, 150, 100, 75, 60, and 50 (Fig. 2.14). Note where the next R wave falls in relation to the six dark vertical lines already marked. This is the heart rate.

Method 3: Small Boxes

The small box method of rate determination is also called *the rule of 1,500*. Each 1-mm box on the graph paper represents 0.04 second. A total of 1,500 boxes represents 1 minute (60 sec/min divided by 0.04 sec/box = 1,500 boxes/min). To calculate the ventricular rate, count the number of small boxes between the R-R interval and divide into 1,500 (see Fig. 2.13). To determine the atrial rate, count the number of small

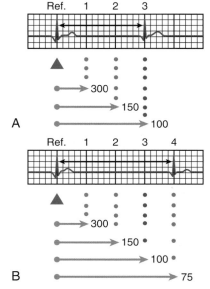

Fig. 2.14 Determining heart rate using the sequence method. To measure the ventricular rate, find a QRS complex that falls on a heavy dark line. Count 300, 150, 100, 75, 60, and 50 until a second QRS complex occurs. This will be the heart rate. (A) Heart rate = 100 beats/min. (B) Heart rate = 75 beats/min. (From Crawford MV, Spence MI: *Commonsense approach to coronary care,* rev ed 6, St. Louis, 1994, Mosby.)

boxes between the P-P interval and divide into 1,500. This method is time consuming but accurate. If the rhythm is irregular, a rate range should be given.

Identify and Examine Waveforms

Look to see if the normal waveforms (P, Q, R, S, and T) are present. To locate P waves, look to the left of each QRS complex. Normally, one P wave precedes each QRS complex (ie, there is a 1:1 relationship); they occur regularly (P-P intervals are equal); and they look similar in size, shape, and position.

Next, evaluate the QRS complex. Are QRS complexes present? If so, does a QRS follow each P wave? Do the QRS complexes look alike? Assess the T waves. Does a T wave follow each QRS complex? Does a P wave follow the T wave? Are the T waves upright and of normal height? Look to see if a U wave is present. If so, note its height and direction (positive or negative).

Assess Intervals and Examine Segments

PR Interval

Intervals are measured to evaluate conduction. Is a PRI present? If so, measure the PRIs and determine if they are equal. The PRI is measured from the point at which the P wave leaves the baseline to the point at which the QRS complex begins. Are the PRIs within normal limits? Remember that a normal PRI measures 0.12 to 0.20 second. If the PRIs are the same, they are said to be constant. If the PRIs are different, is there a pattern? In some dysrhythmias, the duration of the PRI will increase until a P wave appears with no QRS after it. This is referred to as *lengthening* of the PRI. PRIs that vary in duration and have no pattern are said to be *variable*.

QRS Duration

Identify the QRS complexes and measure their duration. The beginning of the QRS is measured from the point at which the first wave of the complex begins to deviate from the baseline. The point at which the last wave of the complex begins to level out, which can be at, above, or below the baseline, marks the end of the QRS complex. The QRS is considered narrow (ie, normal) if it measures 0.11 second or less and wide if it measures more than 0.11 second. A narrow QRS complex is presumed to be supraventricular in origin.

QT Interval

To determine the QT interval, count the number of small boxes between the beginning of the QRS complex and the end of the T wave. Then, multiply that number by 0.04 second. If no Q wave is present, measure the QT interval from the beginning of the R wave to the end of the T wave. The QT interval is prolonged if it is 0.46 second or longer in women or 0.45 second or longer in men.

Examine ST Segments

Determine the presence of ST segment elevation or depression. Remember that the TP segment is used as the baseline from which to evaluate the degree of displacement of the ST segment from the iso-electric line. If ST segment displacement is present, note the number of millimeters of deviation from the J point.

Interpret the Rhythm

Interpret the rhythm, specifying the site of origin (pacemaker site) of the rhythm (sinus), the mechanism (bradycardia), and the ventricular rate (for example, "Sinus bradycardia at 38 beats/min"). Assess the patient to find out how he or she is tolerating the rate and rhythm.

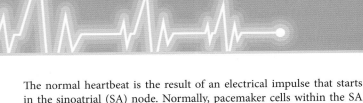

The normal heartbeat is the result of an electrical impulse that starts in the sinoatrial (SA) node. Normally, pacemaker cells within the SA node spontaneously depolarize more rapidly than other cardiac cells. As a result, the SA node usually dominates other areas that may be depolarizing at a slightly slower rate.

A rhythm that begins in the SA node has the following characteristics:

- A positive (ie, upright) P wave before each QRS complex
- P waves that look alike
- A constant PR interval
- A regular atrial and ventricular rhythm (usually)

SINUS RHYTHM

Sinus rhythm is the name given to a normal heart rhythm. Sinus rhythm is sometimes called *regular sinus rhythm* (RSR) or *normal sinus rhythm* (NSR). Sinus rhythm reflects normal electrical activity—that is, the rhythm starts in the SA node and then heads down the normal conduction pathway through the atria, atrioventricular (AV) node and bundle, right and left bundle branches, and Purkinje fibers. In adults and adolescents, the SA node normally fires at a regular rate of 60 to 100 beats/min. A sinus rhythm has the following characteristics:

Rhythm	R-R and P-P intervals are regular
Rate	60 to 100 beats/min
P waves	Positive (upright) in lead II; one precedes each QRS complex; P waves look alike
PR interval	0.12 to 0.20 sec and constant from beat to beat
QRS duration	0.11 sec or less unless abnormally conducted

Fig. 3.1 shows an example of a sinus rhythm recorded simultaneously in three leads: V_1, II, and V_5.

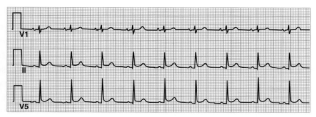

Fig. 3.1 Sinus rhythm with ST segment elevation.

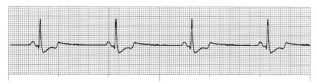

Fig. 3.2 Sinus bradycardia with ST segment depression and inverted T waves.

SINUS BRADYCARDIA

If the SA node fires at a rate slower than normal for the patient's age, the rhythm is called *sinus bradycardia* (Fig. 3.2). The rhythm starts in the SA node and then travels the normal conduction pathway, resulting in atrial and ventricular depolarization. In adults and adolescents, a sinus bradycardia has a heart rate of less than 60 beats/min. The term *severe sinus bradycardia* is sometimes used to describe a sinus bradycardia with a rate of less than 40 beats/min. Sinus bradycardia has the following characteristics:

Rhythm	R-R and P-P intervals are regular
Rate	Less than 60 beats/min
P waves	Positive (upright) in lead II; one precedes each QRS complex; P waves look alike
PR interval	0.12 to 0.20 sec and constant from beat to beat
QRS duration	0.11 sec or less unless abnormally conducted

If a patient presents with a bradycardia, assess how the patient is tolerating the rhythm at rest and with activity. If the patient has no symptoms, no treatment is necessary. The term *symptomatic bradycardia* is used to describe a patient who experiences signs and symptoms of hemodynamic compromise related to a slow heart rate. Treatment of a symptomatic bradycardia should include assessment of the patient's oxygen saturation level and determining if signs of increased work of breathing are present (eg, retractions, tachypnea, paradoxic abdominal breathing). Give supplemental oxygen if oxygenation is inadequate and assist breathing if ventilation is inadequate. Establish intravenous (IV) access and obtain a 12-lead ECG. Atropine, administered intravenously, is the drug of choice for symptomatic bradycardia. Reassess the patient's response and continue monitoring the patient.

SINUS TACHYCARDIA

If the SA node fires at a rate faster than normal for the patient's age, the rhythm is called *sinus tachycardia* (Fig. 3.3). In adults, the rate associated with sinus tachycardia is usually between 101 and 180 beats/min, although faster rates have been documented. Some experts consider the upper rate of sinus tachycardia to be about 220 beats/min, minus the patient's age in years. A sinus tachycardia has the following characteristics:

Rhythm	R-R and P-P intervals are regular
Rate	Usually between 101 and 180 beats/min; alternatively, the upper ventricular rate limit may be calculated as 220 beats/min minus the patient's age in years
P waves	Positive (upright) in lead II; one precedes each QRS complex; P waves look alike
PR interval	0.12 to 0.20 sec and constant from beat to beat
QRS duration	0.11 sec or less unless abnormally conducted

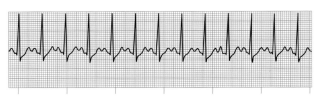

Fig. 3.3 Sinus tachycardia with ST segment depression.

Treatment for sinus tachycardia is directed at correcting the underlying cause (ie, fluid replacement, relief of pain, removal of offending medications or substances, reducing fever or anxiety). Sinus tachycardia in a patient experiencing an acute myocardial infarction (MI) may be treated with medications to slow the heart rate and decrease myocardial oxygen demand (eg, beta-blockers), provided there are no signs of heart failure or other contraindications.

SINUS ARRHYTHMIA

When the SA node fires irregularly, the resulting rhythm is called *sinus arrhythmia* (Fig. 3.4). Sinus arrhythmia that is associated with the phases of breathing and changes in intrathoracic pressure is called *respiratory sinus arrhythmia*. Sinus arrhythmia that is not related to the respiratory cycle is called *nonrespiratory sinus arrhythmia*. Characteristics of sinus arrhythmia include the following:

Rhythm	Irregular and often phasic with breathing; heart rate increases gradually during inspiration (R-R intervals shorten) and decreases with expiration (R-R intervals lengthen)
Rate	Usually 60 to 100 beats/min
P waves	Positive (upright) in lead II; one precedes each QRS complex; P waves look alike
PR interval	0.12 to 0.20 sec and constant from beat to beat
QRS duration	0.11 sec or less unless abnormally conducted

Sinus arrhythmia usually does not require treatment unless it is accompanied by a slow heart rate that causes hemodynamic compromise. If hemodynamic compromise is present as a result of the slow rate, IV atropine may be indicated to treat the bradycardia.

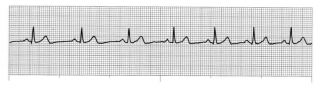

Fig. 3.4 Sinus arrhythmia.

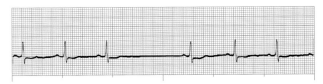

Fig. 3.5 Sinus rhythm with an episode of sinoatrial block.

SINOATRIAL BLOCK

With SA block, also known as *sinus exit block*, the pacemaker cells within the SA node initiate an impulse, but it is blocked as it exits the SA node. This results in periodically absent PQRST complexes (Fig. 3.5). SA block is thought to occur because of failure of the transitional cells in the SA node to conduct the impulse from the pacemaker cells to the surrounding atrium. Characteristics of SA block include the following:

Rhythm	Irregular as a result of the pause(s) caused by the sinoatrial block—the pause is the same as, or an exact multiple of, the distance between two other P-P intervals
Rate	Usually normal but varies because of the pause
P waves	Positive (upright) in lead II; P waves look alike; when present, one precedes each QRS complex
PR interval	0.12 to 0.20 sec and constant from beat to beat
QRS duration	0.11 sec or less unless abnormally conducted

Signs and symptoms associated with SA block depend on the number of sinus beats blocked. If the episodes of SA block are transient and there are no significant signs or symptoms, the patient is observed. If signs of hemodynamic compromise are present and are the result of medication toxicity, the offending agents should be withheld. If the episodes of SA block are frequent, IV atropine, temporary pacing, or insertion of a permanent pacemaker may be needed.

SINUS ARREST

With sinus arrest, the pacemaker cells of the SA node fail to initiate an electrical impulse for one or more beats resulting in absent PQRST complexes on the ECG (Fig. 3.6). When the SA node fails to initiate an

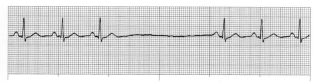

Fig. 3.6 Sinus rhythm with an episode of sinus arrest.

impulse, an escape pacemaker site (eg, the AV junction or the Purkinje fibers) should assume responsibility for pacing the heart. If an escape pacemaker site does not fire, you will see absent PQRST complexes on the ECG. The following are characteristics of sinus arrest:

Rhythm	Irregular; the pause is of undetermined length, more than one PQRST complex is missing, and it is not the same distance as other P-P intervals
Rate	Usually normal but varies because of the pause
P waves	Positive (upright) in lead II; P waves look alike; when present, one precedes each QRS complex
PR interval	0.12 to 0.20 sec and constant from beat to beat
QRS duration	0.11 sec or less unless abnormally conducted

If the episodes of sinus arrest are transient and there are no significant signs or symptoms, observe the patient. If hemodynamic compromise is present, IV atropine, temporary pacing, or both may be indicated. If the episodes of sinus arrest are frequent and prolonged (ie, more than 3 seconds) or a result of disease of the SA node, insertion of a permanent pacemaker is generally warranted.

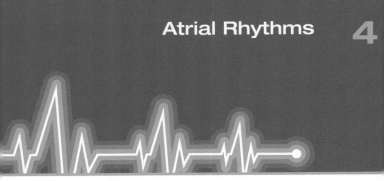

A rhythm that begins in the sinoatrial (SA) node has one positive (ie, upright) P wave before each QRS complex. A rhythm that begins in the atria will have a positive P wave that is shaped differently from P waves that begin in the SA node. This difference in P-wave configuration occurs because the impulse begins in the atria and follows a different conduction pathway to the atrioventricular (AV) node.

PREMATURE ATRIAL COMPLEXES

A *premature atrial complex* (PAC) occurs when an irritable site within the atria fires before the next SA node impulse is expected to fire (Fig. 4.1). This interrupts the sinus rhythm. If the irritable site is close to the SA node, the atrial P wave will look very similar to the P waves initiated by the SA node. The P wave of a PAC may be biphasic (ie, partly positive, partly negative), flattened, notched, pointed, or lost in the preceding T wave. Characteristics of PACs include the following:

Rhythm	Irregular because of the early beat(s)
Rate	Usually within normal range, but depends on underlying rhythm
P waves	Premature (occurring earlier than the next expected sinus P wave), positive (upright) in lead II, one before each QRS complex, often differ in shape from sinus P waves—may be flattened, notched, pointed, biphasic, or lost in the preceding T wave
PR interval	May be normal or prolonged depending on the prematurity of the beat
QRS duration	Usually 0.11 sec or less but may be wide (aberrant) or absent, depending on the prematurity of the beat; the QRS of the premature atrial complex (PAC) is similar in shape to those of the underlying rhythm unless the PAC is abnormally conducted

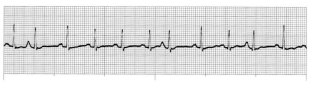

Fig. 4.1 Sinus tachycardia with three premature atrial complexes (PACs). From the left, beats 2, 7, and 10 are PACs.

PAC conducted normally

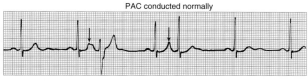

Aberrantly conducted PAC

Fig. 4.2 Premature atrial complexes (PACs) with and without abnormal conduction (aberrancy). (From Kinney MP, Packa DR: *Andreoli's comprehensive cardiac care,* ed 8, St. Louis, 1996, Mosby.)

PACs usually do not require treatment if they are infrequent. The patient may be unaware of their occurrence or, if PACs are frequent, he or she may report feeling a skipped beat or occasional palpitations. In susceptible individuals, frequent PACs may induce episodes of atrial fibrillation (AFib) or paroxysmal supraventricular tachycardia (PSVT). Frequent PACs are treated by correcting the underlying cause. If the patient is symptomatic, frequent PACs may be treated with beta-blockers.

Aberrantly Conducted Premature Atrial Complexes

PACs associated with a wide QRS complex are called *aberrantly conducted PACs.* This indicates that conduction through the ventricles is abnormal (Fig. 4.2).

Nonconducted Premature Atrial Complexes

Sometimes, when a PAC occurs very early and close to the T wave of the preceding beat, a P wave may be seen with no QRS after it (appearing as a pause) (Fig. 4.3). This type of PAC is called a *nonconducted* or *blocked* PAC because the P wave occurred too early to be conducted.

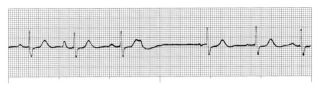

Fig. 4.3 Sinus rhythm with a nonconducted (blocked) premature atrial complex (PAC). Note the distorted T wave of the third QRS complex from the left.

WANDERING ATRIAL PACEMAKER

Multiform atrial rhythm is an updated term for the rhythm formerly known as *wandering atrial pacemaker*. With this rhythm, the size, shape, and direction of the P waves vary, sometimes from beat to beat. The difference in the look of the P waves is a result of the gradual shifting of the dominant pacemaker among the SA node, the atria, and the AV junction (Fig. 4.4). Characteristics of wandering atrial pacemaker include the following:

Rhythm	Usually irregular as the pacemaker site shifts from the SA node to ectopic atrial locations or the AV junction
Rate	Usually 60 to 100 beats/min, but may be slower; if the rate is faster than 100 beats/min, the rhythm is termed *multifocal atrial tachycardia*
P waves	Size, shape, and direction may change from beat to beat; may be upright, inverted, biphasic, rounded, flat, pointed, notched, or buried in the QRS complex
PR interval	Varies as the pacemaker site shifts from the SA node to ectopic atrial locations or AV junction
QRS duration	0.11 sec or less unless abnormally conducted

Wandering atrial pacemaker is usually a transient rhythm that resolves on its own when the firing rate of the SA node increases and the sinus resumes pacing responsibility. If the rhythm occurs because of digitalis toxicity, the drug should be withheld.

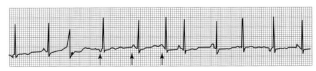

Fig. 4.4 Wandering atrial pacemaker. Note the differences in the shapes of the P waves. (From Paul S, Hebra JD: *The nurse's guide to cardiac rhythm interpretation: Implications for patient care,* Philadelphia, 1998, Saunders.)

MULTIFOCAL ATRIAL TACHYCARDIA

When the wandering atrial pacemaker rhythm is associated with a ventricular rate of more than 100 beats/min, the dysrhythmia is called *multifocal atrial tachycardia* (MAT) (Fig. 4.5). As evidenced by its name, MAT is the result of the random and chaotic firing of multiple ectopic sites in the atria. Characteristics of MAT include the following:

Rhythm	Irregular as the pacemaker site shifts from the SA node to ectopic atrial locations or AV junction
Rate	Faster than 100 beats/min
P waves	One P wave before each QRS but the size, shape, and direction of the P wave may change from beat to beat; may be upright, inverted, biphasic, rounded, flat, pointed, notched, or buried in the QRS complex; at least three different P-wave configurations (seen in same lead) are required for a diagnosis of multifocal atrial tachycardia
PR interval	Varies as the pacemaker site shifts from the SA node to ectopic atrial locations or the AV junction
QRS duration	0.11 sec or less unless abnormally conducted

The treatment of MAT is directed at the underlying cause. If the patient is symptomatic, it is best to consult a cardiologist before starting treatment.

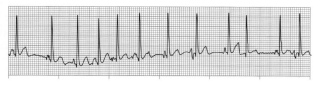

Fig. 4.5 Multifocal atrial tachycardia (MAT). (From Braunwald E, Libby P, Zipes DP, et al: *Heart disease: A textbook of cardiovascular medicine,* ed 6, St. Louis, 2001, Mosby.)

SUPRAVENTRICULAR TACHYCARDIA

Supraventricular arrhythmias begin above the bundle of His; this means that supraventricular arrhythmias include rhythms that begin in the SA node, atrial tissue, or the AV junction. The term *supraventricular tachycardia* (SVT) includes supraventricular rhythms with a ventricular rate faster than 100 beats/min at rest. Three examples of SVTs are shown in Fig. 4.6.

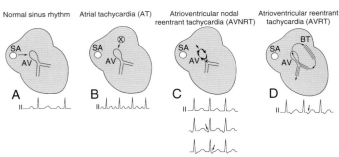

Fig. 4.6 Types of supraventricular tachycardias. A, Normal sinus rhythm is shown here as a reference. B, With atrial tachycardia (AT), a focus (X) outside the sinoatrial (SA) node fires off automatically at a rapid rate. C, With atrioventricular (AV) nodal reentrant tachycardia (AVNRT), the cardiac stimulus originates as a wave of excitation that spins around the AV junctional area. As a result, P waves may be buried in the QRS or appear immediately before or just after the QRS complex (arrows) because of nearly simultaneous activation of the atria and ventricles. D, A similar type of reentrant (circus movement) mechanism in Wolff-Parkinson-White syndrome. This mechanism is referred to as *atrioventricular reentrant tachycardia (AVRT)*. Note the P wave in lead II appears somewhat after the QRS complex. *BT*, bypass tract. (From Goldberger AL: *Clinical electrocardiography: A simplified approach,* ed 7, St. Louis, 2006, Mosby.)

ATRIAL TACHYCARDIA

Atrial tachycardia is a regular rhythm that arises from an ectopic focus in the atria at a rate faster than 100 beats/min and does not require the participation of the AV node to maintain the dysrhythmia (see Fig. 4.6). This rapid atrial rate overrides the SA node and becomes the pacemaker. Characteristics of atrial tachycardia include the following:

Rhythm	Regular
Rate	101 to 250 beats/min
P waves	One P wave precedes each QRS complex in lead II; these P waves differ in shape from sinus P waves; an isoelectric baseline is usually present between P waves; if the atrial rhythm originates in the low portion of the atrium, P waves will be negative in the inferior leads; with rapid rates, it may be difficult to distinguish P waves from T waves

| PR interval | May be shorter or longer than normal; may be difficult to measure because P waves may be hidden in the T waves of preceding beats |
| QRS duration | 0.11 sec or less unless abnormally conducted |

A rhythm that lasts from three beats up to 30 seconds is a *nonsustained rhythm*. A *sustained rhythm* is one that lasts more than 30 seconds. If episodes of AT are short, the patient may be asymptomatic. If AT is sustained and the patient is symptomatic as a result of the rapid rate, treatment should include applying a pulse oximeter and administering oxygen (if indicated), obtaining the patient's vital signs, and establishing IV access. A 12-lead ECG should be obtained. If the patient is not hypotensive, vagal maneuvers may be tried. Although AT will rarely stop with vagal maneuvers, they are used to try to stop the rhythm or slow conduction through the AV node. If vagal maneuvers fail, antiarrhythmic medications should be tried if the patient is hemodynamically stable. If AT is sustained and causing persistent signs of hemodynamic compromise, IV adenosine may be ordered and, if it is ineffective or if administration is not feasible, synchronized cardioversion should be performed.

ATRIOVENTRICULAR NODAL REENTRANT TACHYCARDIA

Atrioventricular nodal reentrant tachycardia (AVNRT) is the most common type of SVT. Patients with AVNRT have two pathways within the AV node that conduct impulses at different speeds and recover at different rates. Under the right conditions, these fast and slow pathways can form an electrical circuit or loop. The result is a very rapid and regular ventricular rhythm (see Fig. 4.6). Characteristics of AVNRT include the following:

Rhythm	Ventricular rhythm is usually very regular
Rate	150 to 250 beats/min; typically 180 to 200 beats/min in adults
P waves	Often hidden in the QRS complex; if the ventricles are stimulated first and then the atria, a negative (inverted) P wave will appear after the QRS in leads II, III, and aVF; when the atria are depolarized after the ventricles, the P wave typically distorts the end of the QRS complex

PR interval	P waves are not seen before the QRS complex; therefore, the PR interval is not measurable
QRS duration	0.11 sec or less unless abnormally conducted

Because AVNRT may be short-lived or sustained, treatment depends on the duration of the tachycardia and severity of the patient's signs and symptoms. If the patient is stable but symptomatic and the symptoms are the result of the rapid heart rate, apply a pulse oximeter and administer supplemental oxygen, if indicated. Obtain the patient's vital signs, establish IV access, and obtain a 12-lead ECG. While continuously monitoring the patient's ECG, attempt a vagal maneuver if there are no contraindications. AVNRT is usually responsive to vagal maneuvers. If vagal maneuvers do not slow the rate or cause conversion of the tachycardia to a sinus rhythm, the first antiarrhythmic given is adenosine. The administration of calcium channel blockers or beta-blockers is indicated when AVNRT fails to convert to sinus rhythm or if it recurs. If the patient is unstable, treatment should include application of a pulse oximeter and administration of supplemental oxygen (if indicated), IV access, and sedation (if the patient is awake and time permits), followed by synchronized cardioversion.

ATRIOVENTRICULAR REENTRANT TACHYCARDIA

Atrioventricular reentrant tachycardia (AVRT) is the next most common type of SVT. The term *preexcitation* is used to describe rhythms that originate from above the ventricles but in which the impulse travels via a pathway other than the AV node and the AV bundle. As a result, the supraventricular impulse excites the ventricles earlier than would be expected if the impulse traveled by way of the normal conduction system (Fig. 4.7). Patients with preexcitation syndromes are prone to AVRT.

The most common form of preexcitation is the Wolff-Parkinson-White (WPW) pattern. The WPW pattern includes a triad of findings that consist of the following: (1) A short PR interval, (2) a delta wave, and (3) a wide QRS complex. A delta wave is an initial slurred deflection at the beginning of the QRS complex that may be positive or negative and reflects the abnormal depolarization of the ventricles through the accessory pathway. A patient is said to have Wolff-Parkinson-White syndrome when a WPW preexcitation pattern is present on the ECG and a tachydysrhythmia occurs that is related to the accessory pathway. Characteristics of WPW syndrome include the following:

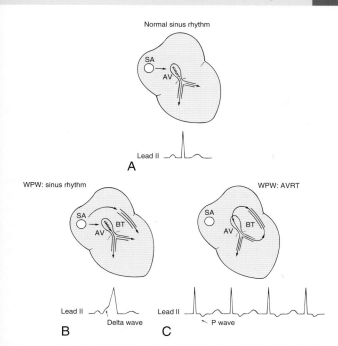

Fig. 4.7 Conduction during sinus rhythm in the normal heart (A) spreads from the sinoatrial (SA) node to the atrioventricular (AV) node and then down the bundle branches. The jagged line indicates physiologic slowing of conduction in the AV node. With Wolff-Parkinson-White (WPW) pattern (B), an abnormal accessory conduction pathway called a bypass tract (BT) connects the atria and ventricles. With WPW, during sinus rhythm, the electrical impulse is conducted quickly down the bypass tract, preexciting the ventricles before the impulse arrives via the AV node. Consequently, the PR interval is short, and the QRS complex is wide, with slurring at its onset (delta wave). WPW predisposes patients to develop an atrioventricular reentrant tachycardia (AVRT) (C) in which a premature atrial beat may spread down the normal pathway to the ventricles, travel back up the bypass tract, and recirculate down the AV node again. This reentrant loop can repeat itself over and over, resulting in a tachycardia. Notice the normal QRS complex and often negative P wave in lead II during this type of bypass-tract tachycardia. (From Goldberger AL: *Clinical electrocardiography: A simplified approach,* ed 7, St. Louis, 2006, Mosby.)

Rhythm	Regular, unless associated with AFib
Rate	Usually 60 to 100 beats/min, if the underlying rhythm is sinus in origin
P waves	Normal and positive in lead II unless Wolff-Parkinson-White syndrome is associated with AFib

PR interval	If P waves are observed, 0.12 sec or less, because the impulse travels very quickly across the accessory pathway, bypassing the normal delay in the AV node
QRS duration	Usually more than 0.12 sec; slurred upstroke of the QRS complex (delta wave) may be seen in one or more leads

Consultation with a cardiologist is recommended when caring for a patient with AVRT.

ATRIAL FLUTTER

Atrial flutter is a reentrant rhythm in which an irritable site within the atria fires regularly at a very rapid rate (Fig. 4.8). Typical atrial flutter is caused by reentry in which an impulse circles around a large area of tissue, such as the entire right atrium, in a counterclockwise direction. Atrial waveforms are produced that resemble the teeth of a saw or a picket fence; these are called *flutter waves* or *F waves*. F waves are predominantly negative in leads II, III, and aVF and positive in V_1. With atypical atrial flutter, the impulse circulates in a clockwise direction, resulting in F waves that are predominantly positive in leads II, III, and aVF and negative in V_1. Characteristics of atrial flutter include the following:

Rhythm	Atrial regular; ventricular regular or irregular depending on AV conduction and blockade
Rate	The atrial rate typically ranges from 240 to 300 beats/min; the ventricular rate varies and is determined by AV blockade; the ventricular rate will usually not exceed 180 beats/min as a result of the intrinsic conduction rate of the AV junction
P waves	No identifiable P waves; saw-toothed flutter waves are present
PR interval	Not measurable
QRS duration	0.11 sec or less but may be widened if flutter waves are buried in the QRS complex or if abnormally conducted

It is best to consult a cardiologist when considering treatment options. If atrial flutter is associated with a rapid ventricular rate and the patient is stable but symptomatic, treatment is usually aimed at controlling the ventricular rate with medications such as beta-blockers (eg, esmolol, metoprolol, propranolol) or nondihydropyridine calcium

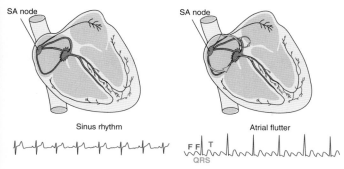

Fig. 4.8 Atrial flutter. *F*, flutter wave.

channel blockers (eg, verapamil, diltiazem). Synchronized cardioversion should be considered for any patient with atrial flutter who has serious signs and symptoms because of the rapid ventricular rate.

ATRIAL FIBRILLATION

AFib occurs because of abnormal automaticity in one or several rapidly firing sites in the atria or reentry involving one or more circuits in the atria (Fig. 4.9). Irritable sites in the atria fire at a rate of 300 to 600 times per minute. These rapid impulses cause the muscles of the atria to quiver (ie, fibrillate), thereby resulting in ineffectual atrial contraction, decreased stroke volume, a subsequent decrease in cardiac output, and a loss of atrial kick. Characteristics of AFib include the following:

Rhythm	Ventricular rhythm usually irregularly irregular
Rate	Atrial rate usually 300 to 600 beats/min; ventricular rate variable
P waves	No identifiable P waves, fibrillatory waves present; erratic, wavy baseline
PR interval	Not measurable
QRS duration	0.11 sec or less unless abnormally conducted

Treatment decisions are based on the ventricular rate, the duration of the rhythm, the patient's general health, and how he or she is tolerating the rhythm. It is best to consult a cardiologist when considering

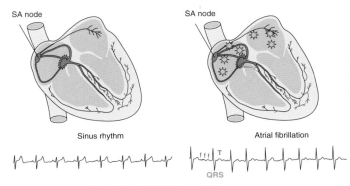

Fig. 4.9 Atrial fibrillation. *f,* Fibrillatory wave.

specific therapies. Rate control and rhythm control are the two primary treatment strategies used to control symptoms of AFib. With rate control, the patient remains in AFib, but the ventricular rate is controlled to decrease acute symptoms, reduce signs of ischemia, and reduce or prevent signs of heart failure from developing. With rhythm control, sinus rhythm is reestablished.

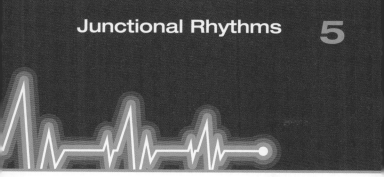

If the atrioventricular (AV) junction paces the heart, the electrical impulse must travel in a backward (*retrograde*) direction to activate the atria (Fig. 5.1). If a P wave is seen, it will be inverted in leads II, III, and aVF because the impulse is traveling away from the positive electrode.

If the atria depolarize before the ventricles, an inverted P wave will be seen *before* the QRS complex, and the PR interval will usually measure 0.12 second or less (Fig. 5.2). The PR interval is shorter than usual because an impulse that begins in the AV junction does not have to travel as far to stimulate the ventricles. If the atria and ventricles depolarize at the same time, a P wave will not be visible because it will be

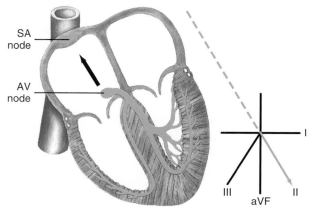

Fig. 5.1 If the atrioventricular (AV) junction paces the heart, the electrical impulse must travel in a backward (retrograde) direction to activate the atria. *SA,* sinoatrial. (From Grauer K: *A practical guide to ECG interpretation,* ed 2, St. Louis, 1998, Mosby.)

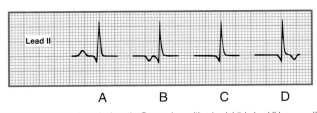

Fig. 5.2 A, With a sinus rhythm, the P wave is positive (upright) in lead II because the wave of depolarization is moving toward the positive electrode. The P wave associated with a junctional beat (in lead II) may be B, inverted (retrograde) and appear before the QRS, C, be hidden by the QRS, or D, appear after the QRS. (From Grauer K: *A practical guide to ECG interpretation,* ed 2, St. Louis, 1998, Mosby.)

hidden in the QRS complex. When the atria are depolarized after the ventricles, the P wave typically distorts the end of the QRS complex and an inverted P wave will appear *after* the QRS. The QRS duration associated with a rhythm that begins in the AV junction measures 0.11 second or less if conduction through the bundle branches, Purkinje fibers, and ventricles is normal.

PREMATURE JUNCTIONAL COMPLEXES

A *premature junctional complex* (PJC) occurs when an irritable site within the AV junction fires before the next sinoatrial (SA) node impulse is ready to fire. This interrupts the sinus rhythm. Because the impulse is conducted through the ventricles in the usual manner, the QRS complex will usually measure 0.11 second or less. Examples of PJCs are shown in Fig. 5.3. Characteristics of PJCs include the following:

Rhythm	Irregular because of the premature beats
Rate	Usually within normal range, but depends on underlying rhythm
P waves	May occur before, during, or after the QRS; if visible, the P wave is inverted in leads II, III, and aVF
PR interval	If a P wave occurs before the QRS, the PR interval will usually be 0.12 sec or less; if no P wave occurs before the QRS, there will be no PR interval
QRS duration	0.11 sec or less unless abnormally conducted

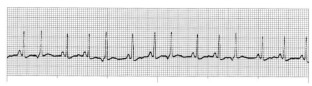

Fig. 5.3 Sinus tachycardia with frequent premature junctional complexes.

PJCs do not normally require treatment because most individuals who have PJCs are asymptomatic. However, PJCs may lead to symptoms of palpitations or the feeling of skipped beats. Lightheadedness, dizziness, and other signs of decreased cardiac output can occur if PJCs are frequent. If PJCs occur because of ingestion of stimulants or digitalis toxicity, these substances should be withheld.

JUNCTIONAL ESCAPE BEATS/RHYTHM

A junctional escape beat begins in the AV junction and appears *late* (ie, after the next expected sinus beat). Junctional escape beats frequently occur during episodes of sinus arrest or follow pauses of nonconducted premature atrial complexes (PACs). An example of a junctional escape beat is shown in Fig. 5.4. Characteristics include the following:

Rhythm	Irregular because of *late* beats
Rate	Usually within normal range, but depends on underlying rhythm
P waves	May occur before, during, or after the QRS; if visible, the P wave is inverted in leads II, III, and aVF
PR interval	If a P wave occurs before the QRS, the PR interval will usually be 0.12 sec or less; if no P wave occurs before the QRS, there will be no PR interval
QRS duration	0.11 sec or less unless abnormally conducted

A junctional *rhythm* is several sequential junctional escape *beats*. The terms *junctional rhythm* and *junctional escape rhythm* are used interchangeably. Remember that the intrinsic rate of the AV junction is 40 to 60 beats/min. Because a junctional rhythm starts from above the ventricles, the QRS complex is usually narrow, and its rhythm is very regular. An example of a junctional rhythm is shown in Fig. 5.5. The ECG characteristics of a junctional rhythm include the following:

Rhythm	Very regular
Rate	40 to 60 beats/min
P waves	May occur before, during, or after the QRS; if visible, the P wave is inverted in leads II, III, and aVF
PR interval	If a P wave occurs before the QRS, the PR interval will usually be 0.12 sec or less; if no P wave occurs before the QRS, there will be no PR interval
QRS duration	0.11 sec or less unless abnormally conducted

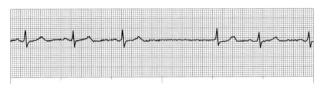

Fig. 5.4 Sinus rhythm with an episode of sinus arrest and a junctional escape beat. (From Aehlert B: *ECG study cards,* St. Louis, 2004, Mosby.)

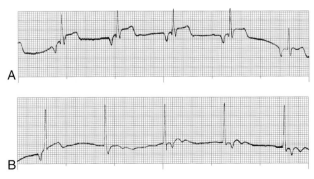

Fig. 5.5 Junctional escape rhythm. Continuous strips. A, Note the inverted (retrograde) P waves before the QRS complexes. B, Note the change in the location of the P waves. In the first beat, the retrograde P wave is seen before the QRS. In the second beat, no P wave is seen. In the remaining beats, the P wave is seen after the QRS complexes. (From Aehlert B: *ECG study cards,* St. Louis, 2004, Mosby.)

The patient may be asymptomatic with a junctional escape rhythm, or he or she may experience signs and symptoms that may be associated with the slow heart rate and decreased cardiac output. Treatment depends on the cause of the dysrhythmia and the patient's presenting signs and symptoms. If the dysrhythmia is caused by digitalis toxicity, this medication should be withheld. If the patient's signs and symptoms are related to the slow heart rate, treatment should include application of a pulse oximeter and administration of supplemental oxygen, if indicated. Establish intravenous (IV) access and obtain a 12-lead ECG. Atropine, given IV, is typically the first medication given for symptomatic bradycardia.

ACCELERATED JUNCTIONAL RHYTHM

If the AV junction speeds up and fires at a rate of 61 to 100 beats/min, the resulting rhythm is called an *accelerated junctional rhythm*. An example of an accelerated junctional rhythm is shown in Fig. 5.6. The ECG characteristics of this rhythm include the following:

Rhythm	Very regular
Rate	61 to 100 beats/min
P waves	May occur before, during, or after the QRS; if visible, the P wave is inverted in leads II, III, and aVF
PR interval	If a P wave occurs before the QRS, the PR interval will usually be 0.12 sec or less; if no P wave occurs before the QRS, there will be no PR interval
QRS duration	0.11 sec or less unless abnormally conducted

The patient is usually asymptomatic because the ventricular rate is 61 to 100 beats/min; however, the patient should be monitored closely. If the rhythm is caused by digitalis toxicity, this medication should be withheld.

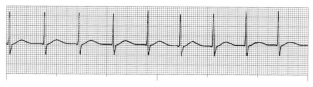

Fig. 5.6 Accelerated junctional rhythm.

JUNCTIONAL TACHYCARDIA

Junctional tachycardia is an ectopic rhythm that begins in the pacemaker cells found in the bundle of His. When three or more sequential PJCs occur at a rate of more than 100 beats/min, a junctional tachycardia exists. Junctional tachycardias can be regular or irregular with variable conduction to the atria.

Nonparoxysmal (ie, gradual onset) *junctional tachycardia* is a benign dysrhythmia that is usually associated with a gradual increase in rate (ie, a warm-up pattern) to more than 100 beats/min. It rarely exceeds 120 beats/min. *Paroxysmal junctional tachycardia*, also known as *focal* or *automatic junctional tachycardia*, is an uncommon dysrhythmia that starts and ends suddenly and is often precipitated by a PJC. The ventricular rate for paroxysmal junctional tachycardia is generally faster, at a rate of 140 beats/min or more. When the ventricular rate is greater than 150 beats/min, it is difficult to distinguish junctional tachycardia from other supraventricular tachycardias. An example of junctional tachycardia is shown in Fig. 5.7. The ECG characteristics of junctional tachycardia include the following:

Rhythm	Ventricular rhythm may be regular or irregular
Rate	101 to 180 beats/min
P waves	May occur before, during, or after the QRS; if visible, the P wave is inverted in leads II, III, and aVF
PR interval	If a P wave occurs before the QRS, the PR interval will usually be 0.12 sec or less; if no P wave occurs before the QRS, there will be no PR interval
QRS duration	0.11 sec or less unless abnormally conducted

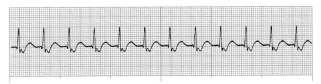

Fig. 5.7 Junctional tachycardia.

Treatment depends on the severity of the patient's signs and symptoms, and expert consultation is advised. If the patient is symptomatic because of the rapid rate, initial treatment should include application of a pulse oximeter and administration of supplemental oxygen, if indicated. Establish IV access and obtain a 12-lead ECG. Because it is often difficult to distinguish junctional tachycardia from other narrow-QRS tachycardias, vagal maneuvers and, if necessary, IV adenosine may be ordered to help determine the origin of the rhythm. If the rhythm is the result of digitalis toxicity, the medication should be withheld. A beta-blocker or calcium channel blocker may be ordered (if no contraindications exist) to slow conduction through the AV node and thereby slow the ventricular rate.

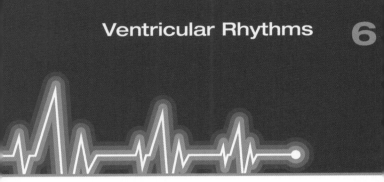

Ventricular Rhythms

6

When an ectopic site within a ventricle assumes responsibility for pacing the heart, the electrical impulse bypasses the normal intraventricular conduction pathway. This results in stimulation of the ventricles at slightly different times. As a result, ventricular beats and rhythms usually have QRS complexes that are abnormally shaped and longer than normal (eg, greater than 0.11 sec). If the atria are depolarized after the ventricles, retrograde P waves may be seen.

Because ventricular depolarization is abnormal, ventricular repolarization is also abnormal and results in changes in ST segments and T waves. The T waves are usually in a direction opposite that of the QRS complex; if the major QRS deflection is negative, the ST segment is usually elevated and the T wave is positive (ie, upright). If the major QRS deflection is positive, the ST segment is usually depressed, and the T wave is usually negative (ie, inverted). P waves are usually not seen with ventricular dysrhythmias, but if they are visible, they have no consistent relationship to the QRS complex.

PREMATURE VENTRICULAR COMPLEXES

A *premature ventricular complex* (PVC) arises from an irritable site within either ventricle. By definition, a PVC is *premature*, occurring earlier than the next expected sinus beat. The shape of the QRS of a PVC depends on the location of the irritable focus within the ventricles (Fig. 6.1). The width of the QRS of a PVC is typically 0.12 sec or greater because the PVC causes the ventricles to fire prematurely and in an abnormal manner (Fig. 6.2). The T wave usually moves in a direction

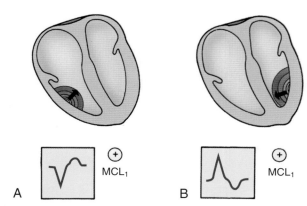

Fig. 6.1 A, Right premature ventricular complex (PVC). The spread of depolarization is from right to left, away from the positive electrode in lead V_1 (MCL$_1$), resulting in a wide, negative QRS complex. B, Left ventricular PVC. The spread of depolarization is from left to right, toward the positive electrode in lead V_1 (MCL$_1$). The QRS complex is wide and upright. (From Urden LD, Stacy KM, Lough ME: *Critical care nursing,* ed 7, St. Louis, 2014, Mosby.)

opposite that of the QRS complex. The general characteristics of PVCs include the following:

Rhythm	Irregular because of the premature beats; if the PVC is an interpolated PVC, the rhythm will be regular
Rate	Usually within normal range, but depends on the underlying rhythm
P waves	Usually absent or, with retrograde conduction to the atria, may appear after the QRS (usually upright in the ST segment or T wave)
PR interval	None with the PVC because the ectopic beat originates in the ventricles
QRS duration	Usually 0.12 sec or greater; T wave is usually in the opposite direction of the QRS complex

Most patients experiencing PVCs do not require treatment with antiarrhythmic medications; rather, treatment of PVCs focuses on the search for, and treatment of, potentially reversible causes. For example, provide reassurance to the patient who is complaining of palpitations

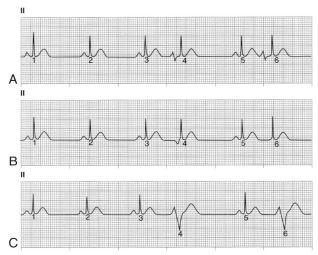

Fig. 6.2 Premature beats. A, Sinus rhythm with premature atrial complexes (PACs). The fourth and sixth beats are preceded by premature P waves that look different from the normally conducted sinus beats. Note that the QRS complex that follows each of these PACs is narrow and identical in appearance to that of the sinus-conducted beats. B, Sinus rhythm with premature junctional complexes (PJCs). The fourth and sixth beats are PJCs. Beat No. 4 is preceded by an inverted P wave with a short PR interval. There is no identifiable atrial activity associated with beat No. 6. C, Sinus rhythm with premature ventricular complexes (PVCs). The fourth and sixth beats are very different in appearance from the normally conducted sinus beats. Beats no. 4 and 6 are PVCs. They are not preceded by P waves. (From Grauer K: *A practical guide to ECG interpretation,* ed 2, St. Louis, 1998, Mosby.)

while searching for possible triggers for his or her PVCs (eg, excessive caffeine ingestion, nicotine use, emotional stress).

VENTRICULAR ESCAPE BEATS/RHYTHM

A ventricular escape beat occurs after a pause in which a supraventricular pacemaker failed to fire; thus, the escape beat is *late*, appearing after the next expected sinus beat. A ventricular escape beat is a *protective* mechanism, safeguarding the heart from more extreme slowing or even asystole. An example of a ventricular escape beat is

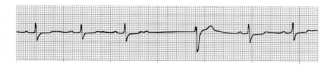

Fig. 6.3 Sinus rhythm with a prolonged PR interval, nonconducted premature atrial complex, ventricular escape beat, and ST-segment depression. (From Chou T, Ramaiah LS: *Electrocardiography in clinical practice: Adult and pediatric,* ed 4, Philadelphia, 1996, Saunders.)

shown in Fig. 6.3. Characteristics of ventricular escape beats include the following:

Rhythm	Irregular because of *late* beats; the ventricular escape beat occurs *after* the next expected sinus beat
Rate	Usually within normal range, but depends on the underlying rhythm
P waves	Usually absent or, with retrograde conduction to the atria, may appear after the QRS (usually upright in the ST segment or T wave)
PR interval	None with the ventricular escape beat because the ectopic beat originates in the ventricles
QRS duration	0.12 sec or greater; the T wave is frequently in the opposite direction of the QRS complex

An *idioventricular rhythm (IVR)*, also known as a *ventricular escape rhythm*, exists when three or more ventricular escape beats occur in a row at a rate of 20 to 40 beats/min. The QRS complexes seen in IVR are wide and bizarre because the impulses begin in the ventricles, bypassing the normal conduction pathway. When the ventricular rate slows to less than 20 beats/min, some practitioners refer to the rhythm as an *agonal rhythm* or *dying heart*. An example of IVR is shown in Fig. 6.4. Characteristics of this rhythm include the following:

Rhythm	Ventricular rhythm is essentially regular
Rate	Ventricular rate 20 to 40 beats/min
P waves	Usually absent or, with retrograde conduction to the atria, may appear after the QRS (usually upright in the ST segment or T wave)
PR interval	None
QRS duration	0.12 sec or greater; the T wave is frequently in the opposite direction of the QRS complex

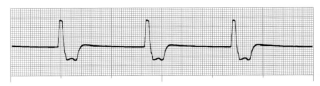

Fig. 6.4 Idioventricular rhythm. (From Aehlert B: *ECG study cards,* St. Louis, 2004, Mosby.)

If the patient has a pulse and is symptomatic because of the slow rate, treatment should include application of a pulse oximeter and administration of supplemental oxygen if indicated. Establish intravenous (IV) access and obtain a 12-lead ECG. Because the ventricular rate is slow, IV atropine may be ordered. Reassess the patient's response and continue monitoring the patient. Transcutaneous pacing or a dopamine or epinephrine IV infusion may be tried if atropine is ineffective. If the patient is not breathing and has no pulse despite the appearance of organized electrical activity on the cardiac monitor, pulseless electrical activity (PEA) exists. The management of PEA should include cardiopulmonary resuscitation (CPR), giving oxygen, starting an IV, possible placement of an advanced airway, and an aggressive search for the underlying cause of the situation.

ACCELERATED IDIOVENTRICULAR RHYTHM

An *accelerated idioventricular rhythm* (AIVR) exists when three or more ventricular beats occur in a row at a rate of 41 to 100 beats/min (Fig. 6.5). AIVR is usually considered a benign escape rhythm that appears when the sinus rate slows and disappears when the sinus rate speeds up. The ECG characteristics of AIVR include the following:

Rhythm	Ventricular rhythm is essentially regular
Rate	41 to 100 (41 to 120 per some cardiologists) beats/min
P waves	Usually absent or, with retrograde conduction to the atria, may appear after the QRS (usually upright in the ST segment or T wave)
PR interval	None
QRS duration	0.12 sec or greater; the T wave is frequently in the opposite direction of the QRS complex

AIVR generally requires no treatment because the rhythm is protective and often transient, spontaneously resolving on its own.

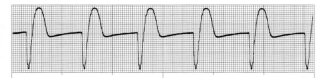

Fig. 6.5 Accelerated idioventricular rhythm. (From Aehlert B: *ECG study cards,* St. Louis, 2004, Mosby.)

VENTRICULAR TACHYCARDIA

Ventricular tachycardia (VT) exists when three or more sequential PVCs occur at a rate of more than 100 beats/min. VT may occur as a short run that lasts less than 30 seconds and spontaneously ends (ie, *nonsustained VT*). *Sustained VT* persists for more than 30 seconds and may require therapeutic intervention to terminate the rhythm. VT may occur with or without pulses, and the patient may be stable or unstable with this rhythm.

Monomorphic Ventricular Tachycardia

When the QRS complexes of VT are of the same shape and amplitude, the rhythm is called *monomorphic VT* (Fig. 6.6). The ECG characteristics of monomorphic VT include the following:

Rhythm	Ventricular rhythm is essentially regular
Rate	101 to 250 (121 to 250 per some cardiologists) beats/min
P waves	Usually not seen; if present, they have no set relationship with the QRS complexes that appear between them at a rate different from that of the VT
PR interval	None
QRS duration	0.12 sec or greater; often difficult to differentiate between the QRS and T wave

Treatment is based on the patient's signs and symptoms and the type of VT. If the rhythm is monomorphic VT (and the patient's symptoms are caused by the tachycardia):

- CPR and defibrillation are used to treat the pulseless patient with VT.
- Stable but symptomatic patients are treated with oxygen (if indicated), IV access, and ventricular antiarrhythmics (eg, procainamide, amiodarone, sotalol) to suppress the rhythm. Procainamide

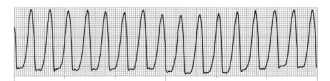

Fig. 6.6 Monomorphic ventricular tachycardia. (From Aehlert B: *ECG study cards,* St. Louis, 2004, Mosby.)

should be avoided if the patient has a prolonged QT interval or signs of heart failure. Sotalol should also be avoided if the patient has a prolonged QT interval.

- Unstable patients (usually a sustained heart rate of 150 beats/min or more) are treated with oxygen, IV access, and sedation (if the patient is awake and time permits) followed by synchronized cardioversion.

In all cases, an aggressive search must be made for the cause of the VT.

Polymorphic Ventricular Tachycardia

With *polymorphic ventricular tachycardia* (PMVT), the QRS complexes vary in shape and amplitude from beat to beat and appear to twist from upright to negative or from negative to upright and back, resembling a spindle. PMVT is a dysrhythmia of intermediate severity between monomorphic VT and ventricular fibrillation (VF) (Fig. 6.7). Several types of PMVT and their possible causes have been identified.

Polymorphic VT has the following ECG characteristics:

Rhythm	Ventricular rhythm may be regular or irregular
Rate	Ventricular rate 150 to 300 beats/min; typically 200 to 250 beats/min
P waves	None
PR interval	None
QRS duration	0.12 sec or more; there is a gradual alteration in the amplitude and direction of the QRS complexes; a typical cycle consists of 5 to 20 QRS complexes

It is best to seek expert consultation when treating the patient with PMVT because of the diverse mechanisms of PMVT for which there may or may not be clues as to its specific cause at the time of the patient's presentation. In general, if the patient is symptomatic as a result of the

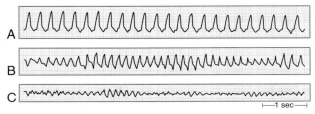

Fig. 6.7 Ventricular tachydysrhythmias. A, Rhythm strip showing monomorphic ventricular tachycardia. B, Example of polymorphic ventricular tachycardia. C, Example of ventricular fibrillation. All tracings are from lead V$_1$. (From Goldman L, Ausiello DA, Arend W, et al: *Cecil medicine,* ed 23, Philadelphia, 2007, Saunders.)

tachycardia, treat ischemia (if it is present), correct electrolyte abnormalities, and discontinue any medications that the patient may be taking that prolong the QT interval. If the patient is stable, the use of IV amiodarone (if the QT interval is normal), magnesium, or beta-blockers may be effective, depending on the cause of the PMVT. If the patient is unstable or has no pulse, proceed with defibrillation as for VF.

VENTRICULAR FIBRILLATION

VF is a chaotic rhythm that begins in the ventricles. In VF, there is no organized depolarization of the ventricles. The ventricular muscle quivers, and as a result, there is no effective myocardial contraction and no pulse. The resulting rhythm looks chaotic with deflections that vary in shape and amplitude (see Fig. 6.7). No normal-looking waveforms are visible. The ECG characteristics of VF include the following:

Rhythm	Rapid and chaotic with no pattern or regularity
Rate	Cannot be determined because there are no discernible waves or complexes to measure
P waves	Not discernible
PR interval	Not discernible
QRS duration	Not discernible

The priorities of care in cardiac arrest as a result of pulseless VT or VF are high-quality CPR and defibrillation. Administer medications and perform additional interventions in accordance with current resuscitation guidelines.

ASYSTOLE

Asystole, also called *cardiac standstill*, is a total absence of atrial and ventricular electrical activity (Fig. 6.8). There is no atrial or ventricular rate or rhythm, no pulse, and no cardiac output. If atrial electrical activity is present, the rhythm is called *P wave asystole* or *ventricular standstill*. Characteristics of asystole include the following:

Rhythm	Ventricular not discernible; atrial may be discernible
Rate	Ventricular not discernible, but atrial activity may be observed (ie, P-wave asystole)
P waves	Usually not discernible
PR interval	Not measurable
QRS duration	Absent

When asystole is observed on a cardiac monitor, confirm that the patient is unresponsive and has no pulse, and then begin high-quality CPR. Additional care includes establishing vascular access, considering the possible causes of the arrest, and administering medications and performing additional interventions in accordance with current resuscitation guidelines.

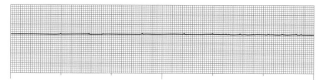

Fig. 6.8 Asystole.

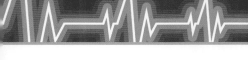

Atrioventricular Blocks 7

7

OVERVIEW

When impulse conduction from the atria to the ventricles is delayed or interrupted because of a transient or permanent anatomic or functional impairment in the conduction system, the resulting dysrhythmia is called an *atrioventricular (AV) block*. When analyzing a rhythm strip, you can assess PR intervals to detect AV conduction disturbances.

AV block is classified into (1) first-degree AV block, (2) second-degree AV block (types I and II), and (3) third-degree AV block. With first-degree AV block, impulses from the sinoatrial (SA) node to the ventricles are *delayed*; they are not blocked. With second-degree AV blocks, there is an *intermittent* disturbance in the conduction of impulses between the atria and the ventricles. With third-degree AV block, there is a *complete* block in the conduction of impulses between the atria and the ventricles.

First-degree AV block usually occurs because of a conduction delay within the AV node (Fig. 7.1). Second- and third-degree AV blocks can occur at the level of the AV node, the bundle of His, or the bundle branches. AV blocks located at the bundle of His or bundle branches are called *infranodal* or *subnodal AV blocks*.

FIRST-DEGREE ATRIOVENTRICULAR BLOCK

With a first-degree AV block, all components of the cardiac cycle are usually within normal limits with the exception of the PR interval. This is because electrical impulses travel normally from the SA node through the atria, but there is a delay in impulse conduction, usually at the level of the AV node (Fig. 7.2). Despite its name, the SA node impulse is not blocked during a first-degree AV block; rather, each sinus impulse is *delayed* for the same period before it is conducted to the ventricles.

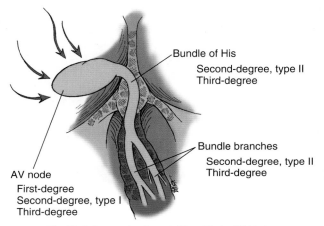

Fig. 7.1 Common locations of atrioventricular (AV) blocks.

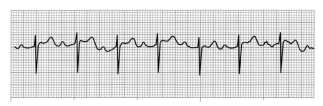

Fig. 7.2 Sinus rhythm with a first-degree atrioventricular block and ST-segment elevation.

Delayed AV conduction results in a PR interval that is longer than normal (ie, more than 0.20 second in duration in adults) and constant PR interval before each QRS complex. The electrocardiogram (ECG) characteristics of first-degree AV block include the following:

Rhythm	Regular
Rate	Usually within normal range, but depends on underlying rhythm
P waves	Normal in size and shape; one positive (upright) P wave before each QRS
PR interval	Prolonged (ie, more than 0.20 sec) but constant
QRS duration	Usually 0.11 sec or less unless abnormally conducted

Patients with first-degree AV block are often asymptomatic. First-degree AV block that occurs with acute myocardial infarction (MI) should be monitored closely to detect progression to higher-degree AV block. If first-degree AV block accompanies a symptomatic bradycardia, treat the bradycardia.

SECOND-DEGREE ATRIOVENTRICULAR BLOCKS

The term *second-degree AV block* is used when one or more, but not all, sinus impulses are blocked from reaching the ventricles. Because the SA node is generating impulses in a normal manner, each P wave will occur at a regular interval across the rhythm strip (ie, all P waves will plot through on time), although not every P wave will be followed by a QRS complex. This suggests that the atria are being depolarized normally, but not every impulse is being conducted to the ventricles (ie, intermittent conduction). As a result, more P waves than QRS complexes are seen on the ECG.

Second-degree AV block is classified as type I or type II, depending on the behavior of the PR intervals associated with the dysrhythmia.

Second-Degree Atrioventricular Block Type I

Second-degree AV block type I is also known as *type I block, Mobitz I,* or *Wenckebach*. With type I AV block, atrial impulses arrive earlier and earlier during the relative refractory period of the AV node, resulting in longer and longer conduction delays and PR intervals, until an impulse arrives during the absolute refractory period and fails to conduct. The nonconducted impulse appears on the ECG as a P wave with no QRS complex after it (Fig. 7.3). ECG characteristics of second-degree AV block type I include the following:

Rhythm	Ventricular irregular; atrial regular (ie, P waves plot through on time); grouped beating may be present
Rate	Atrial rate is greater than the ventricular rate
P waves	Normal in size and shape; some P waves are not followed by a QRS complex (ie, more P waves than QRS complexes)
PR interval	Lengthens with each cycle (although lengthening may be very slight), until a P wave appears without a QRS complex; the PR interval after a nonconducted P wave is shorter than the interval preceding the nonconducted beat
QRS duration	Usually 0.11 sec or less; complexes are periodically dropped

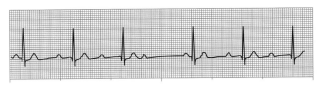

Fig. 7.3 Second-degree atrioventricular block type I.

The patient with type I AV block is usually asymptomatic because the ventricular rate often remains nearly normal, and cardiac output is not significantly affected. If the heart rate is slow and serious signs and symptoms occur because of the slow rate, treatment should include applying a pulse oximeter and administering oxygen (if indicated), obtaining the patient's vital signs, and establishing intravenous (IV) access. A 12-lead ECG should be obtained. Atropine, administered intravenously, is the drug of choice.

Second-Degree Atrioventricular Block Type II

Second-degree AV block type II is also called *type II block* or *Mobitz II AV block*. The site of block in second-degree AV block type II is almost always below the AV node. Although second-degree AV block type II is less common than type I, type II is more serious and is a cause for concern because it has a greater potential to progress to a third-degree AV block. An example of second-degree AV block type II is shown in Fig. 7.4. Characteristics of second-degree AV block type II include the following:

Rhythm	Ventricular irregular; atrial regular (ie, P waves plot through on time)
Rate	Atrial rate is greater than the ventricular rate; ventricular rate is often slow
P waves	Normal in size and shape; some P waves are not followed by a QRS complex (ie, more P waves than QRS complexes)
PR interval	Within normal limits or prolonged but constant for the conducted beats; the PR intervals before and after a blocked P wave are constant
QRS duration	Within normal limits if the block occurs above or within the bundle of His; greater than 0.11 sec if the block occurs below the bundle of His; complexes are periodically absent after P waves

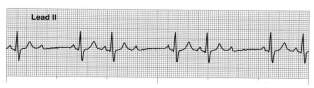

Fig. 7.4 Second-degree atrioventricular block type II. (From Aehlert B: *ECG study cards,* St. Louis, 2004, Mosby.)

Because second-degree AV block type II may abruptly progress to third-degree AV block, the patient should be closely monitored for increasing AV block. If the heart rate is slow and serious signs and symptoms occur because of the slow rate, treatment should include applying a pulse oximeter, obtaining the patient's vital signs, administering oxygen (if indicated), and establishing IV access. A 12-lead ECG should be obtained and a cardiology consult should be sought. Temporary or permanent pacing may be necessary.

2:1 Atrioventricular Block

With 2:1 AV block, there is one conducted P wave followed by a blocked P wave; thus, two P waves occur for every one QRS complex (ie, 2:1 conduction). Because there are no two PQRST cycles in a row from which to compare PR intervals, 2:1 AV block cannot be conclusively classified as type I or type II. To determine the type of block with certainty, it is necessary to continue close ECG monitoring of the patient until the conduction ratio of P waves to QRS complexes changes to 3:2, 4:3, and so on, which would enable PR interval comparison.

If the QRS complex measures 0.11 sec or less, the block is likely to be located in the AV node and a form of second-degree AV block type I (Fig. 7.5). A 2:1 AV block associated with a wide QRS complex (i.e., more than 0.11 sec) is usually associated with a block below the AV node; thus, it is usually a type II block (Fig. 7.6). The ECG characteristics of 2:1 AV block include the following:

Rhythm	Ventricular regular; atrial regular (P waves plot through on time)
Rate	Atrial rate is twice the ventricular rate
P waves	Normal in size and shape; every other P wave is not followed by a QRS complex (ie, more P waves than QRS complexes)
PR interval	Constant
QRS duration	May be narrow or wide; complexes are absent after every other P wave

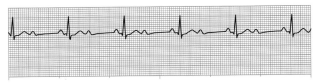

Fig. 7.5 Second-degree 2:1 atrioventricular block with narrow QRS complexes.

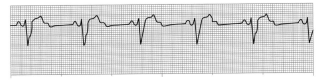

Fig. 7.6 Second-degree 2:1 atrioventricular block with wide QRS complexes.

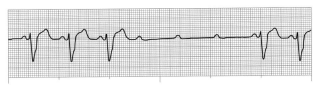

Fig. 7.7 Advanced second-degree atrioventricular block. (From Aehlert B: *ECG study cards,* St. Louis, 2004, Mosby.)

Advanced Second-Degree Atrioventricular Block

The terms *advanced* or *high-grade* second-degree AV block may be used to describe three or more consecutive P waves that are not conducted. For example, with 3:1 AV block, every third P wave is conducted (ie, followed by a QRS complex); with 4:1 AV block, every fourth P wave is conducted (Fig. 7.7).

As is the case with 2:1 AV block, advanced second-degree AV block cannot be conclusively classified as type I or type II because there are no two PQRST cycles in a row from which to compare PR intervals. Monitoring of the patient's ECG for changes in P wave to QRS conduction ratios to enable PR interval comparison is essential. Because of the frequency with which impulses from the SA node to the Purkinje fibers are blocked, the presence of advanced AV block is a cause for concern, and the development of third-degree AV block should be anticipated.

THIRD-DEGREE ATRIOVENTRICULAR BLOCK

With third-degree AV block, the site of block may occur at the level of the AV node, the bundle of His, or distal to the bundle of His (Fig. 7.8). A secondary pacemaker (either junctional or ventricular) stimulates the ventricles; therefore, the QRS may be narrow or wide, depending on the location of the escape pacemaker and the condition of the intraventricular conduction system. The ECG characteristics of third-degree AV block include the following:

Rhythm	Ventricular regular; atrial regular (P waves plot through); no relationship between the atrial and ventricular rhythms (ie, AV dissociation is present)
Rate	The ventricular rate is determined by the origin of the escape pacemaker; the atrial rate is greater than (and independent of) the ventricular rate
P waves	Normal in size and shape; some P waves are not followed by a QRS complex (ie, more P waves than QRS complexes)
PR interval	None; the atria and the ventricles beat independently of each other, so there is no true PR interval
QRS duration	Narrow or wide, depending on the location of the escape pacemaker and the condition of the intraventricular conduction system

The patient's signs and symptoms will depend on the origin of the escape pacemaker (ie, junctional versus ventricular) and the patient's response to a slower ventricular rate. If the patient is symptomatic as a

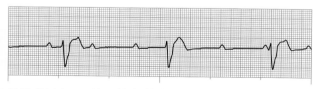

Fig. 7.8 Third-degree atrioventricular block with a wide QRS. (From Aehlert B: *ECG study cards,* St. Louis, 2004, Mosby.)

result of the slow rate, treatment should include applying a pulse oximeter and administering oxygen (if indicated), obtaining the patient's vital signs, establishing IV access, and obtaining a 12-lead ECG. IV administration of atropine may be tried. If the disruption in AV nodal conduction is caused by increased parasympathetic tone, the administration of atropine may be effective in reversing excess vagal tone and improving AV node conduction. Other interventions that may be used in the treatment of third-degree AV block include epinephrine or dopamine IV infusions, or transcutaneous pacing. Frequent patient reassessment is essential. Most patients with third-degree AV block have an indication for permanent pacemaker placement.

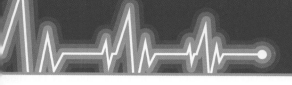

Pacemaker Rhythms 8

INTRODUCTION

A cardiac pacemaker is a battery-powered device that delivers an electrical current to the heart to stimulate depolarization. A pacemaker system consists of a *pulse generator* (ie, the power source) and pacing leads. The pulse generator houses a battery and electronic circuitry. The circuitry works like a computer, converting energy from the battery into electrical pulses. A lithium battery is usually the power source for implanted pacemakers and implantable cardioverter-defibrillators (ICDs), whereas a 9-volt alkaline battery is usually used to power a temporary external pulse generator. A *pacing lead* is an insulated wire used to carry an electrical impulse from the pulse generator to the patient's heart. It also carries information about the heart's electrical activity back to the pacemaker. The pacemaker responds to the information received either by sending a pacing impulse to the heart (ie, *triggering*) or by not sending a pacing impulse to the heart (ie, *inhibition*).

PERMANENT PACEMAKERS AND IMPLANTABLE CARDIOVERTER-DEFIBRILLATORS

A permanent pacemaker is used to treat disorders of the sinoatrial (SA) node (eg, bradycardias), disorders of the atrioventricular (AV) conduction pathways (eg, second-degree AV block type II, third-degree AV block), or both that produce signs and symptoms as a result of inadequate cardiac output. The pacemaker's pulse generator is usually implanted under local anesthesia into the subcutaneous tissue of the anterior chest just below the right or left clavicle.

An ICD is a programmable device that can deliver a range of therapies depending on the dysrhythmia detected and the device programming.

These therapies may include defibrillation, antitachycardia pacing (ie, overdrive pacing), synchronized cardioversion, or bradycardia pacing. A physician determines the appropriate therapies for each patient.

TEMPORARY PACEMAKERS

The pulse generator of a temporary pacemaker is located externally. Temporary pacing can be accomplished through transvenous, epicardial, or transcutaneous means.

Transvenous pacemakers stimulate the endocardium of the right atrium or ventricle (or both) by means of an electrode introduced into a central vein, such as the subclavian, femoral, brachial, internal jugular, or external jugular vein. Epicardial pacing is the placement of pacing leads directly onto or through the epicardium. Epicardial leads may be used when a patient is undergoing cardiac surgery and the outer surface of the heart is easy to reach.

Transcutaneous pacing (TCP) is the use of electrical stimulation through pacing pads positioned on a patient's torso to stimulate contraction of the heart. TCP is indicated for significant bradycardias that are unresponsive to atropine therapy or when atropine is not immediately available or indicated. It may also be used as a bridge until transvenous pacing can be accomplished or the cause of the bradycardia is reversed (eg, drug overdose, hyperkalemia). *Standby pacing* refers to the application of the pacing pads to the patient's chest in anticipation of possible use. For example, standby pacing is often warranted when second-degree AV block type II or third-degree AV block are present in the setting of acute myocardial infarction (MI). The range of output current of a transcutaneous pacemaker varies, depending on the manufacturer.

PACING LEAD SYSTEMS

Pacemaker lead systems may consist of single, double, or multiple leads. The exposed portion of the pacing lead, called an *electrode*, is placed in direct contact with the heart. Pacing, or *pacemaker firing*, occurs when the pacemaker's pulse generator delivers energy (milliamperes [mA]) through the pacing electrode to the myocardium. Evidence of pacing can be seen as a vertical line or spike on the electrocardiogram (ECG).

Capture is the successful conduction of an artificial pacemaker's impulse through the myocardium, resulting in depolarization. Capture is obtained after the pacemaker electrode is properly positioned in the heart; with one-to-one capture, each pacing stimulus results in depolarization of the appropriate chamber. On the ECG, evidence of *electrical capture* can be seen as a pacemaker spike followed by an atrial or ventricular complex, depending on which cardiac chamber is being paced. *Mechanical capture* is assessed by palpating the patient's pulse or by observing right atrial pressure, left atrial pressure, or pulmonary artery or arterial pressure waveforms.

A unipolar electrode has one pacing electrode, which is located at its distal tip. The negative electrode is in contact with the cardiac tissue, and the pulse generator (located outside the heart) functions as the positive electrode. The pacemaker spike produced by a unipolar lead system is often large because of the distance between the positive and negative electrode. Unipolar leads are less commonly used than bipolar lead systems because of the potential for pacing the chest wall muscles and the susceptibility of the unipolar leads to electromagnetic interference.

A bipolar lead system contains a positive and negative electrode at the distal tip of the pacing lead wire. Most temporary transvenous pacemakers use a bipolar lead system. A permanent pacemaker may have either a bipolar or a unipolar lead system. The pacemaker spike produced by a bipolar lead system is smaller than that of a unipolar system because of the shorter distance between the positive and negative electrodes (Fig. 8.1).

PACING CHAMBERS AND MODES

Single-Chamber Pacemakers

A pacemaker that paces a single heart chamber, either the atrium or ventricle, has one lead placed in the heart. Atrial pacing is achieved by placing the pacing electrode in the right atrium. Stimulation of the atria produces a pacemaker spike on the ECG, followed by a P wave (Fig. 8.2). Atrial pacing may be used when the SA node is diseased or damaged, but conduction through the AV junction and ventricles is normal.

Ventricular pacing is accomplished by placing the pacing electrode in the right ventricle. Stimulation of the ventricles produces a pacemaker spike on the ECG followed by a wide QRS, resembling a ventricular ectopic beat (Fig. 8.3). The QRS complex is wide because a paced impulse does not follow the normal conduction pathway in the heart.

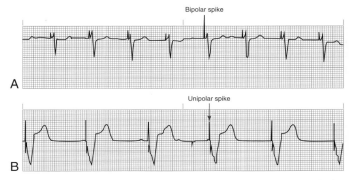

Fig. 8.1 Bipolar and unipolar pacing. A, Pacemaker spike produced by a bipolar lead system. B, Pacemaker spike produced by a unipolar lead system. (From Urden LD, Stacy KM, Lough ME: *Critical care nursing: diagnosis and management,* ed 8, St. Louis, 2018, Mosby.)

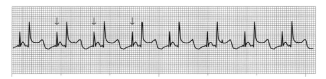

Fig. 8.2 Electrocardiogram of a single-chamber pacemaker with atrial pacing spikes *(arrows).*

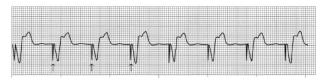

Fig. 8.3 Electrocardiogram of a single-chamber pacemaker with ventricular pacing spikes *(arrows).*

Dual-Chamber Pacemakers

A dual-chamber pacemaker uses two leads; one lead is placed in the right atrium and the other in the right ventricle. Dual-chamber pacing is also called *physiologic pacing.* A dual-chamber pacemaker stimulates the right atrium and right ventricle sequentially (stimulating first the atrium, then the ventricle), mimicking normal cardiac physiology and thus preserving the atrial contribution to ventricular filling (ie, atrial kick) (Fig. 8.4).

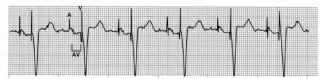

Fig. 8.4 Electrocardiogram of a dual-chamber pacemaker with atrial pacing spikes (A), ventricular pacing spikes (V). *AV*, atrioventricular interval.

Biventricular Pacemakers

A *biventricular pacemaker* has three leads; one lead for each ventricle and one lead for the right atrium. This device uses cardiac resynchronization therapy to restore normal simultaneous ventricular contraction for patients with heart failure, thereby improving cardiac output and exercise tolerance.

Fixed-Rate Pacemakers

A *fixed-rate pacemaker*, also known as an *asynchronous* pacemaker, continuously discharges at a preset rate (usually 70 to 80 impulses/min) regardless of the patient's heart rate or metabolic demands. An advantage of the fixed-rate pacemaker is its simple circuitry, reducing the risk of pacemaker failure; however, this type of pacemaker does not sense the patient's own cardiac rhythm. Fixed-rate pacemakers are not often used today.

Demand Pacemakers

A *demand pacemaker*, also known as a *synchronous* or *noncompetitive* pacemaker, discharges only when the patient's heart rate drops below the pacemaker's base rate. Demand pacemakers can be programmable or nonprogrammable. The voltage level and impulse rate are preset at the time of manufacture in nonprogrammable pacemakers.

PACEMAKER CODES

Pacemaker codes are used to assist in identifying a pacemaker's pre-programmed pacing, sensing, and response functions. The *first letter* of the code identifies the heart chamber (or chambers) paced (stimulated). A pacemaker used to pace only a single chamber is represented by either A (atrial) or V (ventricular). A pacemaker capable of pacing in both chambers is represented by D (dual). The *second letter* identifies the chamber of the heart where patient-initiated (ie, intrinsic) electrical activity is sensed by the pacemaker. The *third letter* indicates how the pacemaker will respond when it senses patient-initiated electrical activity. The *fourth letter* identifies the availability of rate modulation (ie, the pacemaker's ability to adapt its rate to meet the body's needs caused by increased physical activity and then increase or decrease the pacing rate accordingly). A pacemaker's rate modulation capability may also be referred to as *rate responsiveness* or *rate adaptation*. The *fifth letter* denotes multisite pacing.

PACEMAKER MALFUNCTION

Failure to pace is a pacemaker malfunction that occurs when the pacemaker fails to deliver an electrical stimulus at its programmed time. Failure to pace is recognized on the ECG as an absence of pacemaker spikes, even though the patient's intrinsic rate is less than that of the pacemaker, and a return of the underlying rhythm for which pacing was initiated.

Failure to capture is the inability of the artificial pacemaker stimulus to depolarize the myocardium and is recognized on the ECG by visible pacemaker spikes not followed by P waves (if the electrode is located in the atrium) or QRS complexes (if the electrode is located in the right ventricle).

Undersensing occurs when the artificial pacemaker fails to recognize spontaneous myocardial depolarization and is recognized on the ECG by pacemaker spikes that occur within P waves, pacemaker spikes that follow too closely behind the patient's QRS complexes, or pacemaker spikes that appear within T waves. Because pacemaker spikes occur when they should not, this type of pacemaker malfunction may result in pacemaker spikes that fall on T waves (ie, R-on-T phenomenon), competition between the pacemaker and the patient's own cardiac rhythm, or both.

Oversensing is a pacemaker malfunction that results from inappropriate sensing of extraneous electrical signals. Atrial sensing pacemakers may inappropriately sense ventricular activity; ventricular sensing pacemakers may misidentify a tall, peaked, intrinsic T wave as a QRS complex. Oversensing is recognized on the ECG as pacemaker spikes at a rate slower than the pacemaker's preset rate or no paced beats even though the pacemaker's preset rate is greater than the patient's intrinsic rate.

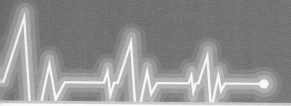

Introduction to the 12-Lead ECG 9

INTRODUCTION

A standard 12-lead electrocardiogram (ECG) provides views of the heart in both the frontal and horizontal planes and views the surfaces of the left ventricle from 12 different angles. Multiple views of the heart can provide useful information including the following:

- Identification of ST-segment and T-wave changes associated with myocardial ischemia, injury, and infarction
- Identification of ECG changes associated with certain medications and electrolyte imbalances
- Recognition of bundle branch blocks

  Indications for using a 12-lead ECG include the following:
- Abdominal/epigastric pain
- Dysrhythmia interpretation
- Chest pain or discomfort
- Diabetic ketoacidosis
- Dizziness
- Dyspnea
- Electrical injuries
- Known or suspected electrolyte imbalances
- Known or suspected medication overdoses
- Right or left ventricular failure
- Status before and after electrical therapy (eg, defibrillation, cardioversion, pacing)
- Stroke
- Syncope or near syncope
- Unstable patient, unknown etiology

VECTORS

Leads have a negative (−) and positive (+) electrode pole that senses the magnitude and direction of the electrical force caused by the spread of waves of depolarization and repolarization throughout the myocardium.

A *vector* (arrow) is a symbol representing this force. A vector points in the direction of depolarization. Leads that face the tip or point of a vector record a positive deflection on ECG paper. A *mean vector* identifies the average of depolarization waves in one portion of the heart. The *mean QRS vector* represents the average magnitude and direction of both right and left ventricular depolarization. The average direction of a mean vector is called the *mean axis*. It is identified only in the frontal plane. An imaginary line joining the positive and negative electrodes of a lead is called the *axis* of the lead. *Electrical axis* refers to the direction, or angle in degrees, in which the main vector of depolarization is pointed.

Axis

Axis determination can provide clues in the differential diagnosis of wide QRS tachycardia and localization of accessory pathways. In adults, the normal QRS axis is considered to be between −30 and +90 degrees in the frontal plane. Current flow to the right of normal is called *right axis deviation* (between +90 and ±180 degrees). Current flow in the direction opposite of normal is called *indeterminate*, "no man's land," *northwest* or *extreme right axis deviation* (−90 and ±180 degrees). Current flow to the left of normal is called *left axis deviation* (between −30 and −90 degrees).

Shortcuts exist to determine axis deviation. Leads I and aVF divide the heart into four quadrants. These two leads can be used to quickly estimate electrical axis. In leads I and aVF, the QRS complex is normally positive. If the QRS complex in either or both of these leads is negative, axis deviation is present.

- Normal axis—positive QRS complex in leads I and aVF
- Right axis deviation—QRS negative in lead I and positive in aVF
- Left axis deviation—QRS positive in lead I and negative in aVF
- Northwest—negative QRS complex in leads I and aVF

ACUTE CORONARY SYNDROMES

Acute coronary syndromes (ACSs) are conditions caused by an abrupt reduction in coronary artery blood flow. Partial or intermittent blockage of a coronary artery may result in no clinical signs and symptoms (silent ischemia), unstable angina (UA), non-ST elevation MI (NSTEMI) or, possibly, sudden death. Complete blockage of a coronary artery may result in ST elevation MI (STEMI) or sudden death. Unstable angina and NSTEMI are often grouped together as *non-ST elevation acute coronary syndromes* (NSTE-ACS) because ECG changes associated with these conditions usually include ST-segment depression and T-wave inversion in the leads that face the affected area. Cardiac biomarkers (eg, troponins) are elevated when an infarction is present. Biomarkers are not elevated in patients with unstable angina because there is no tissue death.

The diagnosis of an ACS is made on the basis of the patient's clinical presentation, history, ECG findings, and cardiac biomarker results. If ST segments are elevated in two contiguous leads and elevated cardiac biomarkers are present, the diagnosis is STEMI. If ST elevation (STE) is not present but biomarker levels are elevated, the diagnosis is NSTEMI. If the ST segments are not elevated and cardiac biomarkers are not elevated, the diagnosis is unstable angina.

When caring for a patient with an ACS, time is muscle. The region of the heart supplied by the blocked artery is called the *area at risk*. The longer the area at risk is deprived of oxygen and nutrients, the greater the likelihood of permanent damage. Therefore, if myocardium is to be saved, the blockage must be removed before irreversible tissue death occurs. If blood flow is quickly restored, the area at risk can potentially be salvaged. The primary choices for reperfusion therapy are fibrinolysis and percutaneous coronary intervention (PCI).

The area supplied by a blocked coronary artery goes through a sequence of events that have been identified as zones of ischemia, injury, and infarction. Each zone is associated with characteristic ECG changes that affect the shape of the QRS complex, the ST segment, and the T wave. ECG changes of myocardial ischemia, injury, or infarction are considered significant if they are viewed in two or more anatomically contiguous leads. If these ECG findings are seen in leads that look directly at the affected area, they are called *indicative changes*. If findings are seen in leads opposite the affected area, they are called *reciprocal changes* (Fig. 9.1).

Leads II, III, and aVF view the inferior wall of the left ventricle. Because these leads "see" the same part of the heart, they are considered contiguous leads. Leads I, aVL, V_5, and V_6 are contiguous because they

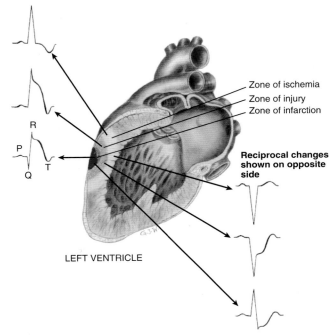

Fig. 9.1 Zones of ischemia, injury, and infarction showing indicative ECG changes and reciprocal changes corresponding to each zone. (Modified from Urden LD, Stacy KM, Lough ME: *Critical care nursing: diagnosis and management,* ed 8, St. Louis, 2018, Mosby.)

all look at adjoining tissue in the lateral wall of the left ventricle. Leads V_1 and V_2 are contiguous because both leads look at the septum. Leads V_3 and V_4 are contiguous because both leads look at the anterior wall of the left ventricle. If right chest leads such as V_4R, V_5R, and V_6R are used, they are contiguous because they view the right ventricle. Leads V_7, V_8, and V_9 are contiguous because they look at the inferobasal (ie, posterior) surface of the heart.

INTRAVENTRICULAR CONDUCTION DELAYS

A *bundle branch block* (BBB) is a disruption in impulse conduction from the bundle of His through either the right or left bundle branch to the Purkinje fibers. A BBB may be intermittent or permanent, complete or incomplete. ECG criteria for BBB recognition include the following:

- QRS duration of 0.12 sec or more in adults (if a *complete* right bundle branch block [RBBB] or left bundle branch block [LBBB]); if a BBB pattern is discernible and the QRS duration is between 0.11 and 0.12 sec in adults, it is called an *incomplete* right or left BBB. (If the QRS is wide but there is no BBB pattern, the term *wide QRS* or *intraventricular conduction delay* is used to describe the QRS).
- Visible QRS complexes produced by supraventricular activity (ie, the QRS complex is not a paced beat, and it does not originate in the ventricles).

If a delay or block occurs in one of the bundle branches, the ventricles will not be depolarized at the same time. The impulse first travels down the unblocked branch and stimulates that ventricle. Because of the block, the impulse must then travel from cell to cell through the myocardium (rather than through the normal conduction pathway) to stimulate the other ventricle. The ventricle with the blocked bundle branch is the last to be depolarized.

With BBB, the last ventricle to be depolarized is the ventricle with the blocked bundle branch. Therefore, if it is possible to determine the ventricle that was depolarized last, it becomes possible to determine the bundle branch that was blocked. The final portion of the QRS complex is referred to as the *terminal force*. Examination of the terminal force of the QRS complex reveals the ventricle that was depolarized last and, therefore, the bundle that was blocked. To identify the terminal force, first locate the J-point. From the J-point, move backward into the QRS and determine if the last electrical activity produced an upward or downward deflection. An example of the terminal force in both RBBB and LBBB is illustrated in Fig. 9.2. If the right bundle branch is blocked, then the right ventricle will be depolarized last, and the current will be moving from the left ventricle to the right. This will create a positive deflection of the terminal force of the QRS complex in V_1. If the left bundle branch is blocked, the left ventricle will be depolarized last, and the current will flow from right to left. This will produce a negative deflection of the terminal force of the QRS complex seen in V_1. Therefore, to differentiate RBBB from LBBB, look at V_1 and determine whether the terminal force of the QRS complex is a positive or negative deflection. If it is directed upward, an RBBB is present (ie, the current is moving toward the right ventricle and toward V_1). An LBBB is present when the terminal force of the QRS complex is directed downward (ie,

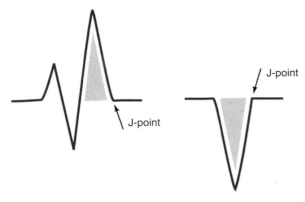

Fig. 9.2 Determining the direction of the terminal force. In lead V_1, move from the J-point into the QRS complex and determine whether the terminal portion (last 0.04 sec) of the QRS complex is a positive (upright) or negative (downward) deflection. (From Phalen T, Aehlert BJ: *The 12-lead ECG in acute coronary syndromes,* ed 3, St. Louis, 2012, Mosby.)

the current is moving away from V_1 and toward the left ventricle). This rule is especially helpful when rSR′ and QS variants are present.

Mike Taigman and Syd Canan have suggested a simple way to remember this rule, demonstrated in Fig. 9.3. They recognized the similarity between this rule and the turn signal on a car. To indicate a right turn, you lift up the arm of the turn signal. Likewise, when an RBBB is present, the terminal force of the QRS complex points up. Conversely, left turns and LBBB move downward.

CHAMBER ENLARGEMENT

Cardiomyopathy is a general term used to describe different types of heart diseases involving the heart muscle and resulting in abnormal enlargement. *Cardiac enlargement* refers to either dilation of a heart chamber or hypertrophy of the heart muscle. With dilation, stretching of a chamber of the heart muscle occurs, resulting in enlargement of that chamber. Dilation may be acute or chronic. *Cardiac hypertrophy* refers to thickening of the heart muscle, with resultant enlargement of a heart chamber. Hypertrophy is commonly accompanied by dilation. When evaluating the ECG for the presence of chamber enlargement, it is particularly important to check the calibration marker to ensure that it is 10-mm (1-mV) tall.

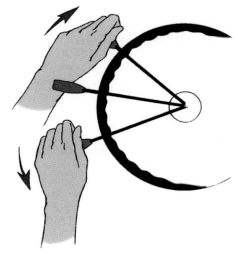

Fig. 9.3 Differentiating between right and left bundle branch blocks. The "turn signal" metaphor helps you remember that right is up and left is down. (From Phalen T, Aehlert BJ: *The 12-lead ECG in acute coronary syndromes,* ed 3, St. Louis, 2012, Mosby.)

Atrial Abnormalities

Right atrial abnormality produces changes in the initial part of the P wave. The P wave is tall (more than 2.5 mm in height), peaked, and usually of normal duration. Lead V_1 may reveal a biphasic P wave. With left atrial abnormality, the middle and end of the P wave is prolonged because depolarization of the left atrium begins and ends later than right atrial depolarization. Notched P waves are usually visible.

Ventricular Abnormalities

Characteristic ECG changes associated with right ventricular hypertrophy include tall R waves in leads V_1 through V_3 and deeper than normal S waves in leads I, aVL, V_5, and V_6. Right axis deviation is usually present, and evidence of right atrial abnormality may be seen. Left ventricular hypertrophy (LVH) is recognized on the ECG by increased QRS amplitude and changes in the ST segment and T wave. Typically, R waves in leads I, aVL, V_5, and V_6 are taller than normal, and S waves in leads V_1 through V_2 are deeper than normal. The QRS duration is often increased.

ELECTROLYTE DISTURBANCES

Because electrolyte imbalances may increase cardiac irritability and cause cardiac dysrhythmias, a patient's ECG can be evaluated for evidence of electrolyte disturbances. It is important to keep in mind that ECG changes associated with electrolyte imbalances can vary widely from patient to patient.

Potassium

Electrocardiographic signs of hyperkalemia can include the following:
- Tall, peaked (tented), narrow, symmetric T waves
- QRS duration increases as potassium level increases
- P waves decrease in amplitude as potassium level increases
- PR interval duration increases as potassium level increases
  Electrocardiographic signs of hypokalemia can include the following:
- ST segment depression
- Decrease in T-wave amplitude
- Prominent U waves; amplitude of U waves may exceed that of T waves in the same lead with marked hypokalemia
- P-wave amplitude and duration are usually increased
- Slight prolongation of PR interval
- Increased QRS duration with severe hypokalemia

Calcium

Electrocardiographic signs of hypercalcemia can include the following:
- Shortening of the ST segment
- Decreased QT-interval duration
  Electrocardiographic signs of hypocalcemia can include the following:
- Lengthening of the ST segment
- Increased QT-interval duration

ANALYZING THE 12-LEAD ELECTROCARDIOGRAM

It is important to use a systematic method when analyzing a 12-lead ECG. Before you begin an in-depth review, pause a moment to take in the entire 12-lead and get an overall impression of the tracing. Does the rate look as if it is normal, fast, or slow? Do the ST segments look markedly elevated or depressed? Is there evidence of premature beats, pauses, baseline wander, or artifact? If baseline wander or artifact is present to any significant degree, note it. If the presence of either of these conditions interferes with the assessment of any lead, use a modifier such as "possible" or "apparent" in your interpretation. After initially surveying the tracing, consider using the following approach when reviewing a 12-lead ECG:

1. Identify the rate and underlying rhythm. Identify any premature beats and pauses, if present.

2. Using lead I and aVF, determine the QRS axis.

3. Identify and examine waveforms and measure intervals. Before examining waveforms, quickly look at the calibration marker and determine if it is standard, half-standard, or twice the standard. Next, examine each lead, selecting one good representative waveform or complex in each lead. Inspect each waveform, noting any changes in orientation, shape, size, and duration.

4. Examine for evidence of ischemia, injury, and infarction. **I See All Leads** is a commonly used mnemonic to recall the lead groupings when localizing an infarction and predicting which coronary artery is occluded. **I** (inferior) = II, III, aVF; **S** (septal) = V_1, V_2; **A** (anterior) = V_3, V_4; **L** (lateral) = I, aVL, V_5, V_6. Look for the presence of ST segment displacement (ie, elevation or depression).

5. Look for evidence of chamber enlargement, look for effects of electrolyte imbalances, and ascertain if conditions that mimic MI are present (eg, LVH, left BBB, ventricular rhythm, ventricular paced rhythm).

Index

Note: Pages followed by "*t*" or "*f*" refer to tables and figures, respectively.